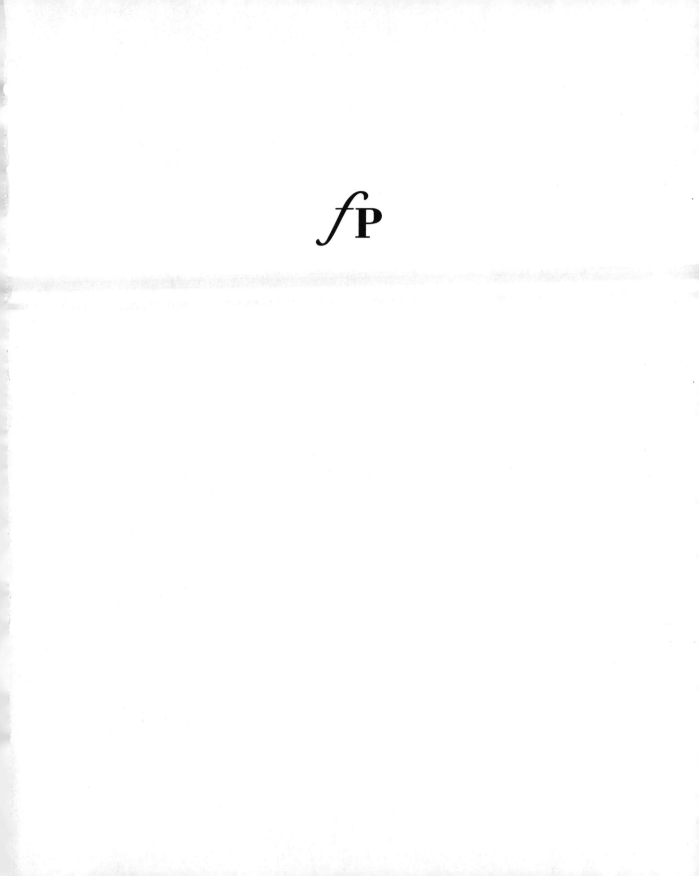

The 17 Day Diet
COOKBOOK

80 All New Recipes for Healthy Weight Loss

DR. MIKE MORENO

FREE PRESS

NEW YORK   LONDON   TORONTO   SYDNEY   NEW DELHI

Note to Readers: This publication is intended to provide helpful and informative material. It is not intended to diagnose, treat, cure, or prevent any health problem or condition, nor is it intended to replace the advice of a physician. No action should be taken solely on the contents of this book. Always consult your physician or qualified health-care professional on any matters regarding your health and before adopting any suggestions in this book or drawing inferences from it.

The author and publisher specifically disclaim all responsibility for any liability, loss, or risk, personal or otherwise, which is incurred as a consequence, directly or indirectly, from the use or application of any contents of this book.

Any and all product names referenced within this book are the trademarks of their respective owners. None of these owners have sponsored, authorized, endorsed, or approved this book. Always read all information provided by the manufacturers' product labels before using their products. The author and publisher are not responsible for claims made by manufacturers. The statements made in this book have not been evaluated by the Food and Drug Administration.

*f*P

FREE PRESS
A Division of Simon & Schuster, Inc.
1230 Avenue of the Americas
New York, NY 10020

Text copyright © 2012 by 17 Day Diet, Inc.
Photographs copyright © 2012 by Nisha Sondhe

First Free Press hardcover edition March 2012

FREE PRESS and colophon are trademarks of Simon & Schuster, Inc.

For information about special discounts for bulk purchases,
please contact Simon & Schuster Special Sales at 1-866-506-1949
or business@simonandschuster.com.

The Simon & Schuster Speakers Bureau can bring authors to your live event.
For more information or to book an event, contact the Simon & Schuster Speakers Bureau
at 1-866-248-3049 or visit our website at www.simonspeakers.com.

Manufactured in the United States of America

10   9   8   7   6   5   4   3   2   1

Library of Congress Cataloging-in-Publication Data is available.

ISBN 978-1-4516-6581-9
ISBN 978-1-4516-6582-6 (ebook)

This book is dedicated to the millions of people who are following the 17 Day Diet to get in shape, reclaim their health, and change their lifestyle for the better.

CONTENTS

ACKNOWLEDGMENTS

As a family practice physician, my passion is, and has always been, to help people take a preventive approach to their health: a full lifestyle change that includes proper diet, regular exercise, and less dependence on prescription drugs. I'm a bit of an exception, rather than the norm, with that lifestyle philosophy. When I designed the 17 Day Diet, I wanted to make sure it supported my prevention philosophy while giving people a program that was sustainable. By all accounts, that goal is being achieved. This cookbook is another tool you can use in your quest for a healthier weight and a healthier life.

I did not put it together on my own. I'd like to thank two superb cooks, Bruce Weinstein and Mark Scarborough, for their contributions. Bruce and Mark grasped the concepts of the diet immediately and were able to turn the 17 Day Diet foods into delicious, easy-to-fix recipes that will become a part of your everyday life. Thanks also to Maggie Greenwood-Robinson for guiding the project, and to the entire amazing team at Free Press, including Leah Miller and Dominick Anfuso, for having the vision and creativity to bring this cookbook about.

INTRODUCTION

Quick show of hands: How many people have rapidly lost a significant amount of weight on the 17 Day Diet? Let's see, that's one, two, three . . . uh, looks like a lot of people.

Now, I'm happy to say that you're going to be able lose even more weight and enjoy it even more with this brand-new cookbook.

Introducing *The 17 Day Diet Cookbook*.

Before you start to panic, rest assured that you don't need to shout and jump and spin knives, make meals that look like a major work of art, or get a degree from Le Cordon Bleu. All you need are some easy-to-follow, easy-to-prepare recipes that are extraordinarily delicious. This cookbook gives you all that and more.

Most of the recipes can be prepared in 30 minutes or less. There are no long lists of ingredients, complicated cooking methods, or hard-to-understand directions. All the recipes are built around the foods you eat on the 17 Day Diet.

The 17 Day Diet is a 4-cycle nutrition program that makes it fast and easy to lose weight, without feeling deprived or hungry all the time. With this companion cookbook, you'll have delectable recipes at your fingertips so you can lose even more weight without giving up delicious foods. It's the perfect way for people with refined palates to lose weight and get healthy. As a family practice physician and an advocate of preventive health, I believe healthy food can still be wonderful. I refuse to accept that a diet has to involve going to extremes or that diet food has to taste like cardboard. It doesn't! It just has to be thoughtfully prepared, in a reasonable amount of time, and taste incredibly good. That's the kind of food you'll find in this book.

I encourage you to try several of these recipes each week to reap the benefits. Broken record, I know, but if you're going to eat healthily and lose more weight, you need to cook more at home. When you do, you have control over what you eat and more control over how much weight you ultimately lose. My nutrition team has developed recipes that taste good and are high in nutrition. We use ingredients that are mainly found in your average grocery store. Use these recipes, and you may never feel like you're on a diet, either!

What I enjoyed most about putting this cookbook together was that I got to sample and test new recipes before they appeared in this book. Some of my favorites are Polynesian London Broil, Tuscan Pork Tenderloin, Crab Cakes, Open-Faced Reuben, Spiced Edamame, Microwaved Mashed Potatoes, Mexican Chocolate Pudding, Chocolaty Frozen Yogurt . . . well, I could go on and on. They're all my favorites!

I'd like to emphasize, too, that cooking at home can also save you a bundle, because you'll likely spend less buying groceries than eating out, and it even can make dating cheaper. After all, who isn't impressed by a partner who knows how to cook? Restaurants must charge high prices in order to pay their employees and other bills. If you cook at home, you design the menu and keep the tips yourself! For health and wealth, there's just no match for a good home-cooked meal, so please start serving more of them.

Home cooking isn't rocket science, either. Lots of us cook and eat. And lots of us love to talk about cooking and eating. We're obsessed with food. With all due respect to baseball, eating is America's real national pastime.

Personally, I just love food. Food and I go way back, more than 43 years now. One of my favorite ways to relax from a day at my office is to come home, roll up my sleeves, and fire up the oven. I'm quite satisfied in the kitchen, experimenting with new recipes, sipping a glass of wine, and enjoying what I've created. And you'll get to enjoy some of these creations right here in this book.

So, if you're in a dietary rut, want to lose even more weight, or are in need of a little inspiration, *The 17 Day Diet Cookbook* is for you!

Refresher Course: The 17 Day Diet

The 17 Day Diet is a 4-cycle program designed to take weight off rapidly. Isn't that what you want? Hardly anyone I know likes to endure depressingly slow weight loss. We want to be trim now, look great now, and feel great now. The 17 Day Diet gets you to where you want to be quickly, without a lot of sacrifice, hunger pangs, or cravings. The diet is nutritionally sound, easy to follow, and it works. I call it the best thing since the sliced bread you'll give up (but only for the first 2 cycles).

Trust me, this is a phenomenal diet. I've had people lose 10 to 12 pounds over the first 17 days, and kept losing steadily right down to their goals. Of course, individuals do vary in their results. The beauty of this program is that you won't get discouraged or bored by the prospect of staying on a diet for what seems like forever because you're shedding fat so quickly. You'll love the fact that in 7, 10, or 17 days, you'll be slimmer. And if your results are like so many others, you'll feel a lot lighter and have an absurd amount of energy.

Overview of the 4 Cycles

The beauty of the 17 Day Diet is that it works in 4 cycles, depending on how much weight you'd like to lose.

Cycle 1 is the initial 17 day period during which you give up all bread, rice, potatoes, pasta, baked goods, fruit, candy, cake, ice cream, and alcohol. It's the strictest period, but also when the most rapid weight loss occurs. And it's easier than you think. You won't even miss carbs after a few days, because your body gets used to not relying on them. You get to eat unlimited amounts of certain proteins and vegetables. And you'll supplement your daily diet with probiotics like yogurt and kefir, foods shown in research to help the body burn fat.

The great thing about Cycle 1 is that you can use it anytime: when you need to break a plateau, get back to your goal weight, fit into a smaller dress size for the weekend or a swimsuit for a cruise, anytime you want to accelerate your weight loss and do it safely. Cycle 1 is one of your best quick-weight loss resources.

During Cycle 2, you slowly begin to reintroduce certain carbs, such as legumes, whole grains, and starchy vegetables, along with lots of other foods. Weight loss continues, and still fairly rapidly. And now, you can drink a little wine, something most diets forbid.

On Cycle 3, you get to eat a huge of array of healthy foods: breads, more meats, more starches, and fun foods like low-carb frozen dessert treats. You ease off some of the strictness of the first 2 cycles, while still continuing to knock off pounds. Every 17 days you're changing things up, so you never get bored. Every day is exciting, because you see the results on your scale or in your more loosely fitting clothes.

Cycle 4 is the maintenance period that, ideally, you stay on the rest of your life. It lets you stay at your new weight as long as you do two things: enjoy yourself on the weekend, and use your favorite cycle during the week. So, once you're happy with your new svelte self, continue to enjoy occasional forbidden foods. Just do so carefully or you'll find yourself back on a slippery slope to your prediet weight. If you fall off the wagon for a weekend or, say, on a vacation, don't panic. Just jump back to Cycle 1 to quickly shave off any weight you gain.

Why the 17 Day Diet Works So Well

Eliminating unhealthy foods from your system keeps them from making a beeline to your belly and elsewhere. Healthy foods do the opposite. The higher amounts of lean protein you eat on this diet, for example, boost your metabolism in a number of physiologically active ways. This diet is high in fiber, too, which is an appetite suppressant, a detoxifier, and a food component that ushers bad calories out of your system before they have time to camp out on your thighs. Then there is the addition of probiotics, now believed to keep fat formation in check.

Another reason that the 17 Day Diet works is because you're changing your calorie count and the foods you eat. By varying these things, you keep your body and metabolism guessing. I call this *body confusion*. The scale is less likely to get stuck. The added bonus: You'll never get bored. And it's fun watching those pounds melt off. So, confusion is good!

But, more important, the 17 Day Diet works because it's realistic and sustainable. Nothing derails a diet faster than distressing round-the-clock hunger pangs, or boredom. But the 17 Day Diet isn't about depriving yourself of food or variety. I encourage you to eat until you are no longer hungry, even snack between meals, as long as you're eating the right foods. That doesn't mean just broccoli, either. Nuts, cheeses, and other delicious foods are permitted as you progress through the cycles. There are so many choices, too, that you'll never get bored.

Let's Start Cooking and Losing

You've read this and you're a believer, and you can't wait to get started. To learn all the intricacies of how and why the diet works, you need to get the book, *The 17 Day Diet*, and its other companion book, *The 17 Day Diet Workbook*. If you can't get to the bookstore right away, here's an overview of the diet:

Quick and Easy Overview of the 17 Day Diet	
Cycle	**Purpose**
Cycle 1: Accelerate (17 days)	To promote rapid weight loss by improving digestive health. This cycle helps clear sugar from the blood to boost fat-burning and discourage fat storage.
Cycle 2: Activate (17 days)	To reset your metabolism through a strategy that involves increasing and decreasing your caloric consumption to stimulate fat-burning, and to help prevent plateaus.

Cycle 3: Achieve (17 days)	To develop good eating habits through the reintroduction of additional foods and move you closer to your goal weight.
Cycle 4: Arrive (ongoing)	To keep you at your goal weight through a program of eating that lets you enjoy your favorite foods on weekends, while eating healthfully during the week.

How to Use This Cookbook

For losing weight on *The 17 Day Diet*, this cookbook is divided into three easy-to-digest sections:

- Cycle 1 Recipes and Cycle 1 17 Day Meal Plan

- Cycle 2 Recipes and Cycle 2 17 Day Meal Plan

- Cycle 3 Recipes and Cycle 3 17 Day Meal Plan

Each section features delicious breakfasts, lunches, dinners, and snacks that match the cycle you're in. I show you how to use those recipes by giving you menu plans for each cycle. That's a total of 51 daily menus to help you.

Follow these delicious meal plans, week by week. They will give you structure, which helps guard against unplanned eating, plus you can learn about some new foods and ways to prepare them. The meal plans are low in fat, high in fiber, packed with nutrition, and designed to trigger rapid weight loss. I strongly believe that the way you eat to control your weight must continue for the rest of your life. These meal plans can help you do that. They provide a lifelong foundation for a healthy, enjoyable, and satisfying way of eating.

Now that you're acquainted with how the 17 Day Diet works in conjunction with this cookbook, it's time to take action. People who have used this plan have told us they could not believe how effortless it was to lose weight and keep it off. Why? Because the 17 Day Diet is a way of life. Unlike your past dieting experiences, you'll never need to quit. As long as you keep going, you'll see results. Beginning in Cycle 1, you'll start to shed unwanted pounds and renew your vitality.

I know you'll enjoy what we've cooked up here. These are recipes that can satisfy your appetite and help you drop pounds. Each one has been created to help you succeed at getting your weight under control without skimping on the flavors you love.

I know you want meals that are quick and healthy. You want them to taste wonderful, you want them to help you lose weight, and you want them now! Seems like a tall order, but that's what these recipes deliver, especially if you're prepared. Just start with a cycle's worth of meals, and do it. Having the right ingredients on hand, plus kitchen equipment that makes preparation easier, will make cooking quicker and more healthful.

Time-savers are built into each recipe, too. For example, they take advantage of healthy convenience foods available in supermarkets, such as boneless, skinless chicken breasts. All you have to do is apply the finishing touches. For side dishes, you'll use quick-cooking staples such as washed greens and salad mixes, frozen fruits and vegetables, and quality convenience products, such as prepared salad dressings and low-calorie condiments.

Preparing the 17 Day Diet recipes requires no special equipment, although some appliances (suggested but not required) can help, and these are listed for you here. There are few meals that can't be made leaner or healthier by using cooking methods such as broiling, steaming, baking, lightly stir-frying, microwaving, and sautéing in water or with vegetable cooking spray. With every new recipe you try, you will discover low-fat and low-carb cooking tips; healthy methods of food preparation; ways to cut the fat, sugar, calories, and cholesterol; and how to use fresh herbs and spices to add flavor. We also include important information on kitchen tools that can help you prepare healthful meals. You may already have a lot of the gear in your kitchen. The rest you should be able to pick up at any kitchenware or houseware store. Consider these tools to help you get your weight under control. The more weight-loss tools you have, the more successful you will be.

Now, the 17 Day Diet recipes. Enjoy!

Pots and Pans

Look for heavy pots and pans, preferably with nonstick coatings and tight-fitting lids. The nonstick coating can help you cut down the amount of oil or other fats you need to coat the pan, and it'll make cleanup a lot easier.

Saucepans: at least three (one 1-quart pan, one 2-quart pan, and one 3-quart pan)
Skillets: two or three (one 7- and/or 8-inch skillet and one 12-inch skillet)
Soup pot: one 5- or 6-quart pot

Utensils

Stocking your kitchen with the following utensils will make your culinary efforts easier and more enjoyable. You may even find that having a couple of sets of some items, such as wooden spoons and spatulas, is more convenient than having to wash the tools several times throughout the preparation of a dish or meal.

Colander
Cutting board
Egg separator
Garlic press
Grater
Kitchen scissors
Spatulas
Strainer
Timer
Whisks
Wooden spoons

Other Useful Items

If you have the storage space in your kitchen, these additional items are less essential, but definitely helpful.

Baking pans: at least one 13- x 9- x 2-inch pan;
at least one 8- x 8- x 2-inch pan

Muffin tin: one or two

Baker's rack: preferably a large, square one, for cooling bread and muffins. A rack permits the air to circulate, reducing sogginess.

Casserole dishes: at least two (one 1½-quart dish and one 3-quart dish), with covers

Mixing bowls: several sizes

Slow cooker (such as a Crock-Pot): good for soups and lean cuts of meats

Steamer rack: for cooking vegetables and reheating foods that do best with moist heat

Wok: for stir-frying and steaming

The 17 Day Diet
COOKBOOK

RECIPES

Cycle 1—Accelerate

GOAL: To trigger rapid weight loss in a healthy manner by mobilizing fat stores and flushing water and toxins from your system.

Snappy Eggs

Skipping breakfast is not a good idea. People who skip breakfast are more likely to overeat at other times throughout the day and gain weight. I realize that you might not have a lot of time in the morning, but here's a recipe that will let you enjoy a great breakfast even if you're crunched for time.

INGREDIENTS
2 cups prepared salsa
4 large eggs

DIRECTIONS

1. Position a rack in the middle of the oven and preheat to 400°F. Spoon the salsa into an 8-inch baking dish. Set in the oven and heat for 15 minutes.

2. Remove the baking dish from the oven. Use the back of a wooden spoon to create 4 evenly spaced wells in the salsa. Crack an egg into each of these wells. Return to the oven and bake until the whites are set but the yolks are still soft, 8 to 10 minutes. (For hard-cooked yolks, bake for 15 minutes.) Use a large spoon to scoop the eggs into serving bowls along with the hot salsa.

YIELD: 2 servings (can be doubled using a 9- x 13-inch baking dish)

> **TIPS:** Heat the salsa while you take a shower! There are lots of salsas on the market so you can customize the eggs to your taste: peach salsa. Extra hot salsa. Experiment!

Spanish Omelet

Being of Hispanic descent, I love fluffy Spanish omelets. Add a couple fresh jalapeno slices for more zip. The eggs whites here cut the fat and calories and also make it a healthy, high-protein dish.

INGREDIENTS
- 1 egg
- 2 egg whites
- ⅛ teaspoon salt
- ⅛ teaspoon black pepper
- 1 tablespoon olive oil
- ¼ cup diced tomato
- 2 tablespoons diced onion
- 2 tablespoons shredded fat-free cheddar cheese

DIRECTIONS

1. In a medium bowl, whisk together egg, egg whites, salt, and black pepper. Heat a frying pan over medium-high heat.

2. Add olive oil and swirl pan to coat bottom and sides. Add eggs and tilt pan to spread mixture across entire pan bottom. Cook for about 30 seconds.

3. With a spatula, gently lift sides of omelet and tilt pan to distribute more uncooked egg to the pan's surface. Once the egg begins to set, sprinkle diced tomato, onion, and cheddar cheese over one side of the omelet. Carefully fold the other side of the omelet over the fillings.

YIELD: 1 serving

Mushroom Spinach Frittata

To me, eggs are everything they're cracked up to be. I absolutely love them in any way, shape, or form. Here's one of my favorite egg recipes. I've had it for breakfast, brunch, lunch, and dinner. If you've never had breakfast for dinner, you have no idea what you're missing!

INGREDIENTS

3 large eggs

2 large egg whites

1 (10 ounces) package frozen chopped spinach, thawed

2 teaspoons olive oil

6 ounces thinly sliced white or cremini mushrooms

1 tablespoon minced fresh oregano leaves or 1 teaspoon dried oregano

½ teaspoon salt

½ teaspoon ground black pepper

½ teaspoon red-pepper flakes, optional

DIRECTIONS

1. Use a fork or a whisk to beat the eggs and egg whites in a small bowl until creamy and thick. Set aside.

2. Squeeze the chopped spinach by handfuls over the sink to remove excess moisture. Set aside.

3. Heat the olive oil in a 10-inch, nonstick skillet over medium heat. Add the mushrooms; cook, stirring often, until they give off some of their liquid and it then evaporates, about 5 minutes.

4. Crumble in the spinach; stir in the oregano, salt, pepper, and red-pepper flakes, infusing. Stir for 2 minutes to warm the spinach and toast the spices.

5. Beat the eggs one more time to make sure they're creamy, then pour them into the skillet. Reduce the heat to low, cover, and cook until set and no longer loose, about 10 minutes. Loosen the frit-

(continued on next page)

Mushroom Spinach Frittata (*cont.*)

tata with a heat-safe rubber spatula and slide onto a cutting board to slice into quarters.

YIELD: 2 servings

> **TIP:** Put the box of frozen chopped spinach in the fridge the night before to thaw.

Greek Egg Scramble

Enjoy this quick-to-fix feast and the flavors—yet another great way to start the day. I love Greek food so much, I should be Greek!

INGREDIENTS

Nonstick cooking spray

4 egg whites

¾ cup chopped red onions

¼ cup diced tomato

2 tablespoons crumbled reduced-fat feta cheese

⅛ teaspoon salt

⅛ teaspoon black pepper

DIRECTIONS

1. In a medium bowl, combine all ingredients.

2. Pour into a small frying pan that has been coated with nonstick spray.

3. Cook over medium-low heat 2 to 3 minutes, stirring frequently, until eggs are cooked through.

YIELD: 1 serving

Peach Melba Smoothie

Smoothies are a great way to sneak your fruit in, and give you plenty of nourishing vitamins, minerals, and phytochemicals *(plant chemicals that contain protective, disease-preventing compounds). Whenever I crave something sweet, I go for a smoothie because it's perfectly satisfying and I feel totally energized afterward. This recipe is a spectacular combination; hardly anything so nutritious tastes this good.*

INGREDIENTS

2 cups plain, low-fat, unsweetened kefir

1 medium peach, peeled, pitted and sliced into wedges

1 cup raspberries

1 teaspoon Truvia

⅛ teaspoon ground cinnamon

2 ice cubes

DIRECTIONS

Place all the ingredients in a blender; cover and blend until smooth. Divide into two glasses.

YIELD: 2 servings

> **TIP:** Use 6 ounces frozen peach slices. You can save half the smoothie in a covered container in the fridge, for a snack later. Give it a whirl to make sure it's smooth before serving.

Kefir Smoothie

I like kefir. I've always liked the idea of fermented milk, which is healthy, natural, and beneficial, but had never actually tried the stuff. I always thought it might be too sour for my tastes, so when grocery shopping, I'd always look at it and think, "The kefir looks great," and then grab a quart of chocolate milk. I incorporated kefir into the 17 Day Diet because it's a fat-burning probiotic; now I love it, especially in smoothies.

INGREDIENTS
    1 cup unsweetened kefir
    1 cup frozen unsweetened berries
    1 tablespoon sugar-free fruit jam or 1 tablespoon agave nectar
    1 tablespoon flaxseed oil

DIRECTIONS
Place all ingredients in a blender and blend until smooth.

YIELD: 1 large serving

Yogurt Fruitshake

Don't worry: Acidophilus milk *might sound unappetizing but it tastes just like regular milk. Plus, it gives you a healthy dose of probiotics to help you manage your weight.*

INGREDIENTS
½ cup acidophilus milk
3 ounces sugar-free fruit-flavored yogurt
1 cup frozen unsweetened berries

DIRECTIONS
Place all ingredients in a blender and blend until smooth.

YIELD: 1 large serving

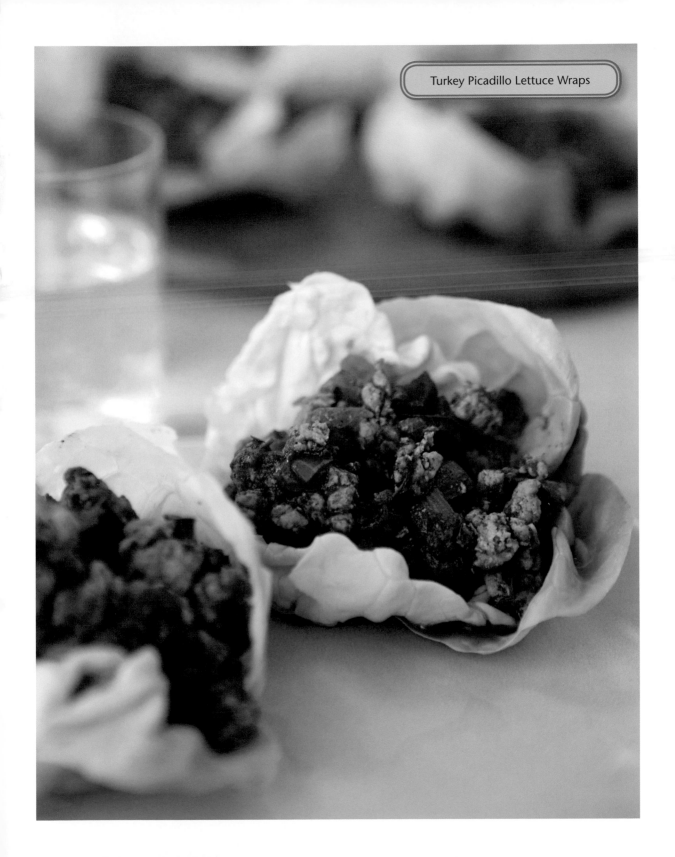

Turkey Picadillo Lettuce Wraps

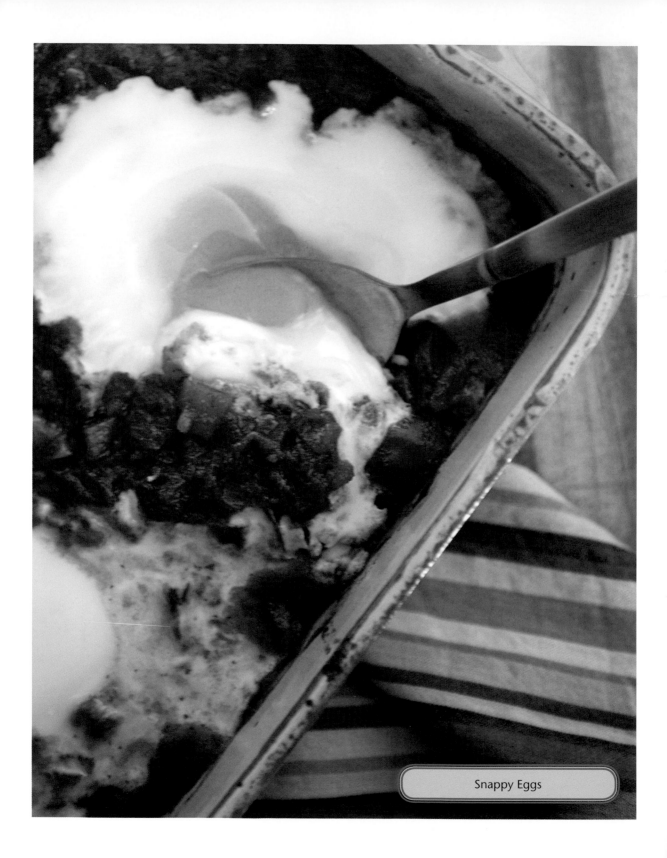

Snappy Eggs

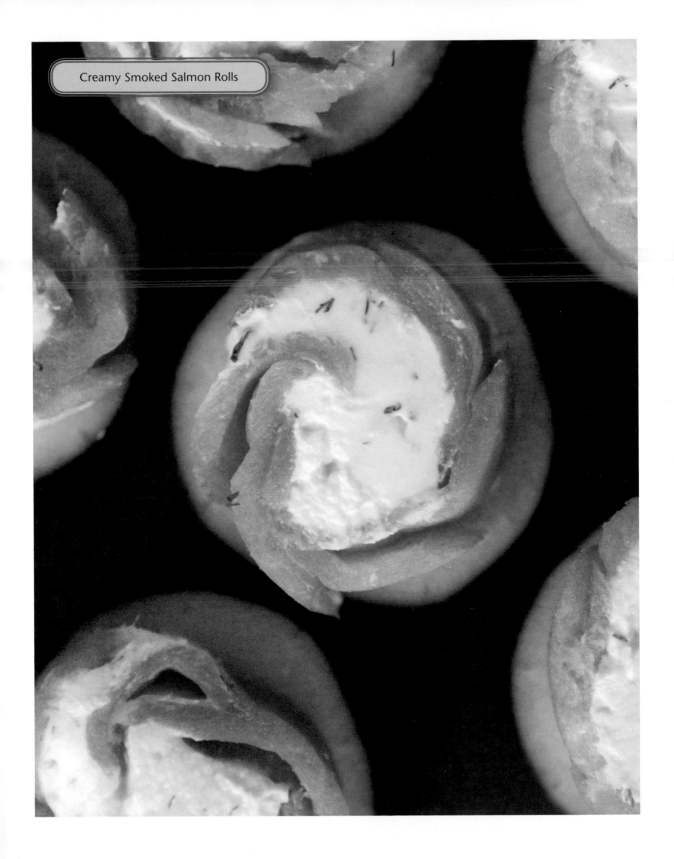
Creamy Smoked Salmon Rolls

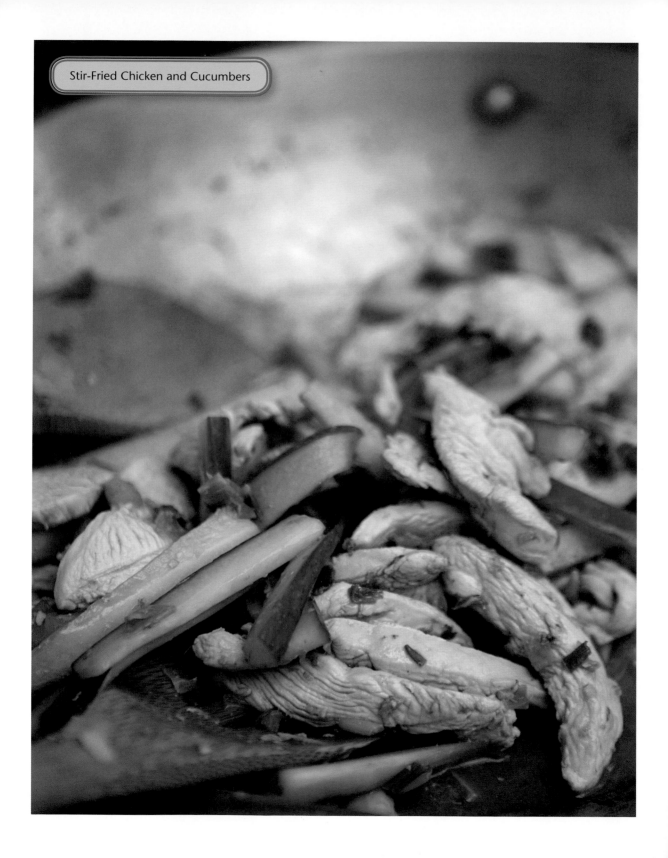

Stir-Fried Chicken and Cucumbers

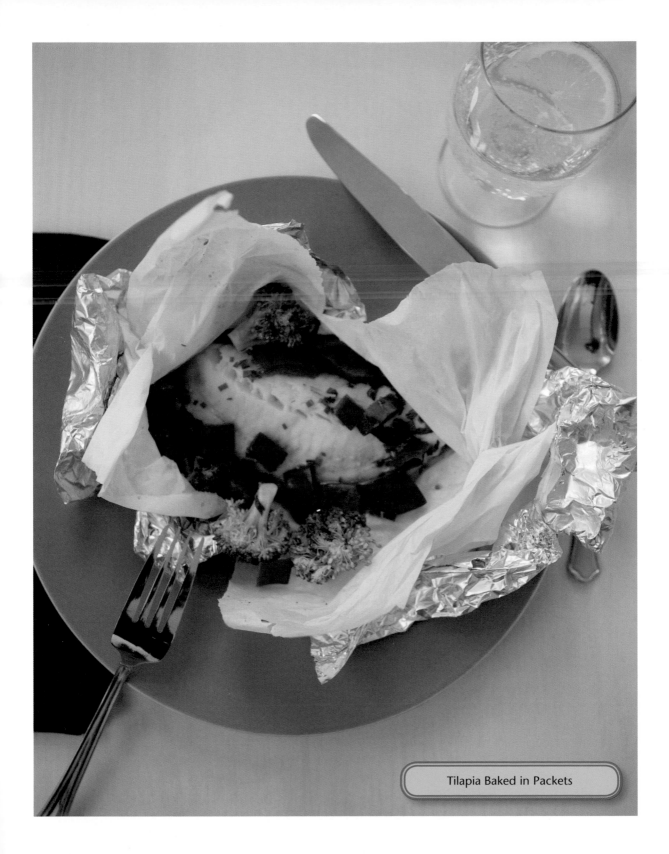

Tilapia Baked in Packets

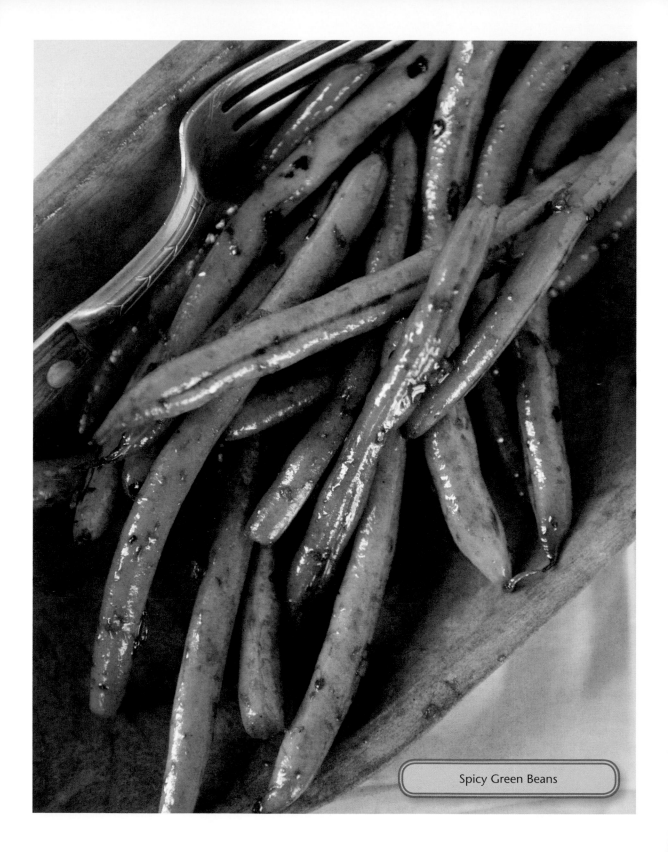

Spicy Green Beans

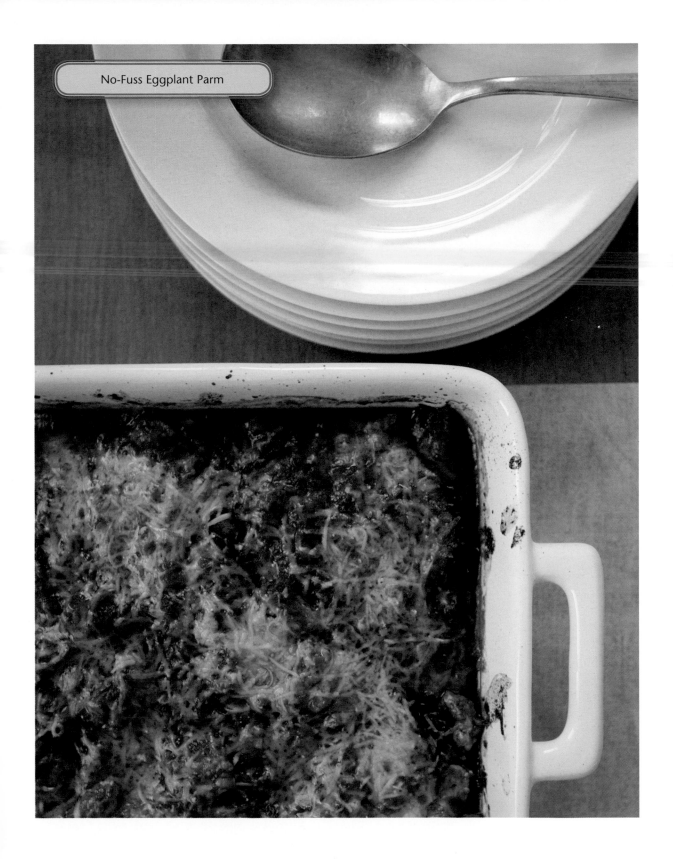

No-Fuss Eggplant Parm

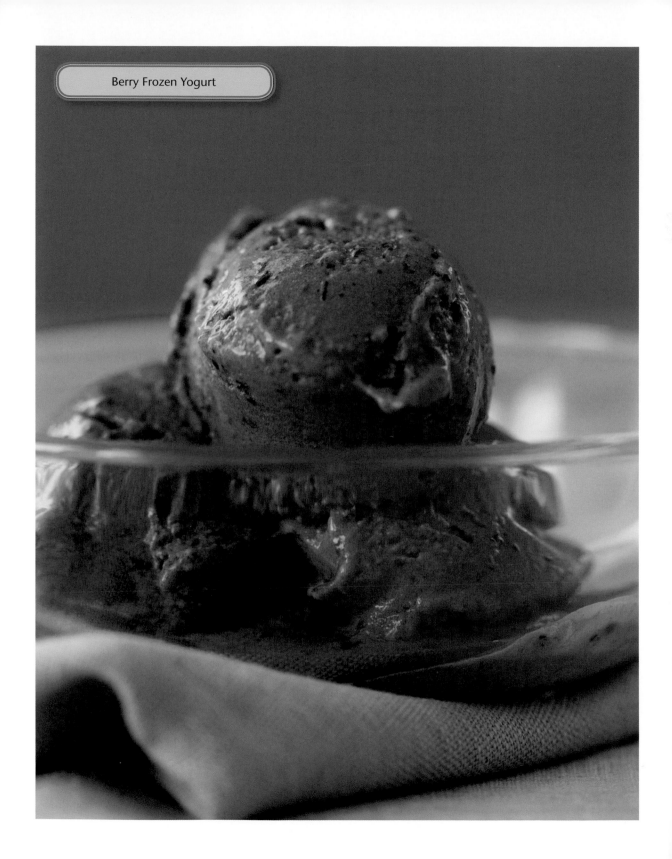

Berry Frozen Yogurt

Chicken-Vegetable Soup

This is a water-based soup, which offers a lot of weight-control benefits, such as helping to control hunger, reducing total calorie intake when eaten before or with a meal, and filling you up. It's also a good source of nutrients you might fall short of.

INGREDIENTS

1½ cups chopped cabbage

1 large carrot, chopped

1 cup sliced okra

1 large onion, chopped

2 large celery stalks with leaves, chopped

1 can (15 ounces) crushed tomatoes

1 can (14 ounces) fat-free chicken broth

1½ teaspoons salt

¼ teaspoon pepper

4 baked boneless, skinless chicken breasts, diced

DIRECTIONS

1. Place all ingredients except chicken in a large pan and simmer for 1 hour, or until vegetables are soft.

2. Add chicken and heat thoroughly.

YIELD: 4 servings

California Tuna Salad

Whether it's piled on top of a salad, stuffed in fresh tomatoes, or slathered between two slices of whole-wheat bread, I love tuna salad. However, it's important to prepare it so that you can control the amount of fat that goes into it. Translation: No creamy mayonnaise smothering the tuna! This version of tuna salad is low in fat, and oh so delicious, as well as easy to fix. Please note: Tuna tends to be high in mercury; however, this recipe uses light canned tuna, which is lower in mercury. My advice is to eat tuna no more than twice a week to be on the cautious side.

INGREDIENTS

- 2 tablespoons lemon juice
- Up to 1½ tablespoons olive oil, optional
- 2 teaspoons Dijon mustard
- ½ teaspoon salt
- ½ teaspoon black pepper
- 1 can (6 ounces) light tuna packed in water, drained
- 1 (8½ ounce) can artichoke hearts packed in water, drained, and halved
- 2 celery stalks, minced
- 2 medium scallions, thinly sliced

DIRECTIONS

Whisk the lemon juice, olive oil, if using, mustard, salt, and pepper in a large bowl until smooth and creamy. Add the remaining ingredients and stir until combined and coated.

YIELD: 2 servings (can be doubled or tripled)

TIPS: Serve on a bed of lettuce. For less fat, omit lemon juice, olive oil, mustard, salt, and pepper; use ¼ cup fat-free, no-carb honey Dijon or creamy Italian dressing, such as Walden Farms dressings. If you love tuna salad, always keep a couple of cans in the refrigerator, so that when you make this salad, it's already cool.

Super Salad

Any diet that leaves you feeling hungry is doomed to fail. The 17 Day Diet will not do that. It's high in foods that make you feel full, like veggies. So have your fill of this salad, and it will keep you feeling full.

INGREDIENTS

Lettuce, any variety, torn into bite-sized pieces

Cucumbers

Onions

Tomatoes

Other salad vegetables, such as celery, bell peppers, or raw broccoli

2 hard-boiled eggs, peeled and chopped

2 tablespoons olive or flaxseed oil

4 tablespoons balsamic vinegar

DIRECTIONS

1. Combine lettuce with vegetables and hard-boiled eggs.

2. Toss with olive or flaxseed oil and balsamic vinegar.

3. Season to taste.

YIELD: 1 serving

Turkey Picadillo Lettuce Wraps

Want a suitable substitute for bread? Try lettuce wraps. They make great sandwiches, they're more filling than bread (because lettuce is high in water volume), and keep your carb intake down to practically zero.

INGREDIENTS

Nonstick cooking spray

1 medium yellow onion, chopped

1 medium garlic clove, minced

1 medium red bell pepper, stemmed and chopped

1 pound lean ground turkey

1 large tomato, roughly chopped

¼ cup minced fresh parsley leaves or 2 tablespoons dried parsley flakes

1 tablespoon minced fresh oregano leaves or 1 teaspoon dried oregano

1 tablespoon chili powder

1 tablespoon Worcestershire sauce

½ teaspoon cinnamon

1½ teaspoons apple-cider vinegar

8 Romaine or Boston lettuce leaves, thick stems removed

DIRECTIONS

1. Spray a large skillet with nonstick cooking spray. Set over medium heat for 1 minute. Add onion and garlic. Cook, stirring occasionally, until softened, about 3 minutes. Add the bell pepper; continue cooking, stirring occasionally, about 2 minutes

2. Add the ground turkey, and break up with a spoon. Cook, stirring frequently, until lightly browned, about 6 minutes.

3. Raise the heat to medium-high. Stir in the tomato, parsley, oregano, chili powder, Worcestershire sauce, and cinnamon. Cook, stirring occasionally, until the tomatoes break down, their liquid evaporates, and the skillet is almost dry, about 5 minutes. Remove from the heat and stir in the vinegar. Cool for 10 minutes, then

spoon a scant ½ cup filling into each lettuce leaf; roll the leaves up, like burritos, and serve.

YIELD: 4 servings

> **TIPS:** For a take-along lunch, pack the picadillo and the lettuce leaves separately. To save prep time, look in the produce section of your supermarket for cut-up bell peppers and even onions.

Lemon-Pepper Salmon Salad in Tomato Cups

This super-low-fat salmon salad with fresh tomatoes looks and is delicious enough to serve when you're entertaining. Don't assume that means being tied up for hours in the kitchen. You can make this salad fast, and ahead of time. And if there's one food I could live on, it's salmon. It's chock-full of omega-3 fatty acids, which are good for brain function and for combating inflammation and stiffness.

INGREDIENTS

1 can (6 ounces) salmon, drained

2 celery stalks, minced

¼ cup fat-free sour cream

2 tablespoons minced yellow onion

1 teaspoon lemon-pepper seasoning

2 large tomatoes

DIRECTIONS

1. Mix the salmon, celery, sour cream, onion, and lemon-pepper seasoning in a small bowl.

2. Slice ¼ inch off the stem end of each tomato. Use a serrated grapefruit spoon or a melon baller to scoop out the seeds and membranes, leaving 2 tomato cups. Spoon half the salmon salad into each cup to serve.

YIELD: 2 servings (can be doubled or tripled)

TIPS: For the best taste, look for wild-caught, skinless, boneless, Alaskan pink salmon. To mince celery, cut the stalks lengthwise into thin strips, then slice these as thin as possible. For a take-along lunch, carry the salad and tomatoes separately. The salad can stay covered in the fridge for up to 3 days, but not in the tomato cups.

Creamy Smoked Salmon Rolls

Bagels are the traditional accompaniment to lox and cream cheese, but since you can't eat bagels until later on the diet, here's an amazing alternative that will satisfy your taste buds while waiting.

INGREDIENTS

- 4 ounces thinly sliced lox or smoked salmon
- ½ cup yogurt cheese made from fat-free, plain Greek yogurt (see recipe below)
- ½ teaspoon fresh dill
- ½ teaspoon finely grated lemon zest
- ¼ teaspoon garlic powder
- 1 large cucumber, sliced into ¼-inch disks

DIRECTIONS

1. Lay a large piece of wax paper on your work surface. Lay the smoked salmon slices on the wax paper, overlapping them to make a large rectangle. Spread the yogurt cheese on top of the salmon; sprinkle evenly with the dill, lemon zest, and garlic powder. Using the wax paper to lift the salmon up, roll the fish like a jelly roll, taking care that the wax paper is only a guide and doesn't get caught inside the roll. Wrap the log in plastic wrap; refrigerate for at least 1 hour or up to 24 hours.

2. Unwrap the roll; lay on a cutting board. Use a serrated knife to slice into ½-inch-thick pinwheels. Place each piece on top of a cucumber disk.

YIELD: 2 servings

> **TIP:** Make ahead, slice off as much of the log as you want, then rewrap the rest of the log and refrigerate.

Yogurt Cheese

This easy-to-make cheese can be enjoyed as a tangy dip for vegetables or, in later cycles, as a topping for baked potatoes. It is completely fat free and tastes just like high-fat sour cream.

INGREDIENTS

32 ounces fat-free Greek yogurt
Spices, such as Kosher salt, garlic, or oregano

DIRECTIONS

1. Line a strainer with a coffee filter or white paper towel. Place the strainer over a bowl to catch the liquid. Spoon in 32 ounces of fat-free plain yogurt.

2. Cover and refrigerate for 8 hours or overnight.

3. Makes about 16 ounces of yogurt cheese. Mix in your favorite spices for a tangy dip for vegetables or as a topping for baked potatoes.

Stir-Fried Chicken and Cucumbers

The best fast food around is stir-fry. Granted, there may be some chopping involved, but that's a small price to pay for a delicious hot meal you can serve this quickly.

INGREDIENTS

Nonstick cooking spray

6 medium scallions, sliced thin

1 tablespoon peeled minced fresh ginger

1 medium garlic clove, minced

1 pound boneless skinless chicken breasts, sliced thin

2 medium cucumbers, halved lengthwise, seeded, and sliced thin

2 tablespoons light soy sauce

2 tablespoons unseasoned rice vinegar

Up to 1 teaspoon hot red-pepper sauce, optional

DIRECTIONS

1. Spray a large wok or skillet with nonstick cooking spray; set over medium-high heat until smoking. Add the scallions, ginger, and garlic. Toss and stir over the heat for 30 seconds.

2. Add the chicken strips. Toss and stir until lightly browned and any trace of pink is gone, about 3 minutes.

3. Add the cucumbers. Stir-fry until heated through and softening at the edges, about 2 minutes. Pour in the soy sauce, rice vinegar, and hot red-pepper sauce, if using. Stir until bubbling, until the chicken has absorbed some of the sauce, less than 1 minute.

YIELD: 4 servings

(continued on next page)

Stir-Fried Chicken and Cucumbers (*cont.*)

LUNCH

TIPS: For an even quicker meal, look in the butcher case for sliced boneless skinless chicken breasts, sometimes sold as chicken breasts for stir-fries.

No need to peel cucumbers if they are organic or from a farmers market. However, most standard cucumbers from the supermarket have been waxed with a food-grade wax and should be peeled for the best-tasting dish.

Rice vinegar needs a note. Unseasoned rice vinegar is just rice vinegar, usually not labeled as anything other than rice vinegar. "Seasoned" rice vinegar includes sugar. Make sure you have unseasoned; look at the ingredient list on the bottle's label.

Hot red-pepper sauce. You can use Tabasco or a similar hot sauce. I really like the Indonesian sambal olek, which is banging hot. It's now available in the Asian section of almost every supermarket.

Tandoori Chicken Breasts

I love Indian food, and this traditional tandoori chicken fills the bill. The chicken is marinated in yogurt and spices, then cooked to perfection. Yogurt, a key fat-burning ingredient in the 17 Day Diet, is very popular in Indian and Middle Eastern cooking, both in sauces and side dishes to help soothe the tongue while eating spicy entrees.

INGREDIENTS

⅓ cup plain, low-fat yogurt or plain, low-fat kefir

1 tablespoon curry powder

½ teaspoon Truvia

¼ teaspoon garlic powder

Nonstick cooking spray

Four 4-ounce boneless skinless chicken breasts

1½ pounds baby spinach leaves, washed but not dried

DIRECTIONS

1. Mix the yogurt, curry powder, Truvia, and garlic powder in a large bowl to make a wet paste. Add the chicken breasts; stir and toss until well coated. Cover and store in the fridge for at least 30 minutes or up to 4 hours.

2. Spray a grill pan with nonstick cooking spray and set over medium-high heat. Alternatively, spray a large baking sheet with nonstick cooking spray, set it on the oven rack 4 to 6 inches from the broiler element, and preheat the broiler.

3. Place the chicken breasts on the grill pan or the baking sheet. (Do not wipe off the marinade.) Grill or broil for 8 minutes, turning once, until browned and cooked through. Transfer the cooked chicken to a cutting board.

4. Dump the wet spinach into a large saucepan and set over medium heat. Cook, tossing often, until the spinach begins to wilt and steam from the moisture, about 2 minutes. Divide the spinach

(*continued on next page*)

Tandoori Chicken Breasts (*cont.*)

among four serving plates. Slice the chicken into strips; fan these out over the spinach.

YIELD: 4 servings

TIPS: This dish can also be served with Oven-Roasted Cauliflower and Broccoli (page 34). Greek yogurt is too thick for this dish. Use regular yogurt or kefir to coat the chicken breasts. There is an astounding array of curry powders on the market, not only the standard, yellow version. Search for big-flavored varieties in the international aisle of most large supermarkets, or look for one to your taste at East Indian supermarkets or online.

Low-Carb Primavera Delight

Who needs carby noodles when you've got spaghetti squash? This low-carb dish will fill you up without filling you out, and you won't even miss the pasta.

INGREDIENTS
    1 spaghetti squash
    2 cups chopped fresh broccoli
    1 small onion, diced
    2 minced garlic cloves
    1 tablespoon olive oil
    Marinara sauce, for serving, heated

DIRECTIONS
1. Preheat the oven to 375 degrees. To prepare the squash, cut it in half. Scoop out the seeds and pulp as you would any squash or pumpkin.

2. Place squash, rind side up, in a glass baking dish filled with about ½ inch of water. Bake 40 to 45 minutes, or microwave the squash for 8 to 10 minutes per half on high.

3. Let the squash stand for a few minutes after cooking. Separate strands by running a fork through it lengthwise. Place strands in a bowl.

4. While squash is cooking, in a medium frying pan set over medium-high heat, cook the broccoli, onion, garlic, and oil until vegetables are crisp-tender, stirring constantly, about 4 minutes. Add squash and heat thoroughly. Serve on plates topped with marinara sauce.

YIELD: 4 servings

No-Fuss Eggplant Parm

Eggplant Parmesan, an Italian standby, is one of my favorite dishes. We developed this quick version so that I could have it more often. It's super low in carbs and fat, and you won't even miss the breading.

INGREDIENTS

Nonstick cooking spray

1 large eggplant, stemmed and sliced into ½-inch-thick rounds

1 pound lean ground turkey

4 cups low-carb prepared marinara sauce

1½ tablespoons minced fresh oregano leaves or 2 teaspoons dried oregano

1 teaspoon fennel seeds

1½ cups grated fat-free cheese, such as Parmesan

DIRECTIONS

1. Position a rack in the center of the oven and preheat to 350°F. Spray a large baking sheet with nonstick cooking spray. Lay the eggplant slices on the baking tray and spray their tops lightly with nonstick cooking spray. Bake, turning once, until the slices begin to soften and brown, about 30 minutes.

2. Meanwhile, spray a large saucepan with nonstick cooking spray. Set over medium heat and add the ground turkey, breaking it up with a spoon. Cook, stirring often, until the meat loses its raw, pink color and browns a bit, about 5 minutes. Pour in the marinara sauce; stir in the oregano and fennel seeds. Remove the pot from the heat.

3. Layer the eggplant slices and turkey marinara sauce in a 9- x 13-inch baking dish. Sprinkle the cheese on top. Bake until bubbling, about 30 minutes. Cool for 5 minutes before serving.

YIELD: 4 servings

Curried Poached Halibut

While grilling, *or holding a chunk of meat above a fire, might be the oldest form of cookery,* poaching, *or cooking in simmering liquid was probably not far behind. For a simple dinner, a poached fillet of fish served with a sauce made by reducing the cooking liquid is fast and easy.*

INGREDIENTS

- 1½ cups fat-free, reduced-sodium chicken broth
- 1 large leek, white and pale green parts only, halved lengthwise, rinsed thoroughly, and sliced thin
- 1 large red bell pepper, stemmed, seeded, and chopped
- 2 cups small cauliflower florets
- 1 tablespoon peeled minced fresh ginger or prepared minced ginger
- 1 tablespoon curry powder
- Four 4-ounce skinless halibut fillets
- ½ cup plain, low-fat yogurt
- 1 teaspoon lemon juice

DIRECTIONS

1. Pour the broth into a large, deep skillet; a wide, deep saucepan; or a Dutch oven. Stir in the leeks, bell pepper, cauliflower, ginger, and curry powder. Set over medium heat; bring to a low simmer. Cover, reduce heat to low, and simmer for 5 minutes.

2. Place the fillets into the broth mixture. Cover and continue simmering until the fish is cooked through and flakes when touched with a fork, 8 to 10 minutes.

3. Use a slotted spoon or a wide spatula to transfer the fish to four serving bowls. Remove the skillet or pan from the heat and stir the yogurt and lemon juice into the sauce. Divide the sauce among the bowls.

(continued on next page)

Curried Poached Halibut (*cont.*)

TIPS: Slice larger cauliflower florets into smaller pieces. Look for prepared minced ginger in the produce section. Don't buy if it is brown; look for beige bits of ginger that have not broken down. Refrigerate for freshness.

Grilled Tuna Niçoise Salad

The Niçoise salad is a French classic from Nice. It's usually made with hard-boiled eggs, anchovies, black olives, tomatoes, and so forth. Our version uses a lot of Cycle 1 veggies instead, to cut the calories but not the flavor.

INGREDIENTS

1 pound tuna steak, about ½ inch thick

2 teaspoons olive oil

½ teaspoon salt

½ teaspoon black pepper

1 pound small cauliflower florets

¾ pound green beans, stemmed and cut into 1-inch pieces

¾ pound small asparagus spears, cut into 1-inch pieces

12 cherry tomatoes, halved

½ cup fat-free, low-carb, bottled French dressing, such as Walden Farms

1 medium head Romaine lettuce, cored, and leaves torn into small pieces

DIRECTIONS

1. Rub the tuna steak with the olive oil on both sides; sprinkle with salt and pepper. Heat a large grill pan over medium-high heat. Add the tuna; cook until medium-rare, about 6 minutes, turning once. (Cook about 8 minutes for well-done.) Transfer to a cutting board.

2. Bring a large saucepan of water to a boil over high heat. Add the cauliflower, green beans, and asparagus. Cook for 3 minutes. Drain in a colander. Rinse with cool water to stop cooking; drain well. Transfer the vegetables to a large bowl.

3. Cut the tuna into pieces about the size of the vegetables; add to the bowl. Add the tomatoes. Add the dressing and toss gently. Divide the Romaine lettuce among four plates; spoon a quarter of the grilled tuna salad on top of the lettuce on each plate.

YIELD: 4 servings

(continued on next page)

Grilled Tuna Niçoise Salad (*cont.*)

TIP: Try using bottled low-carb, fat-free, sugar-free vinaigrette

Oven-Barbecued Chicken

I don't want to incur the wrath of barbecue purists by introducing this quick-to-fix oven version, but I defy you to come away from the table without a glow of satisfied contentment after eating this. The chicken is just a bit sweet, thanks to the wonderful natural sweetener agave nectar with a bit of heat that emphasizes the chicken flavor.

INGREDIENTS

Nonstick cooking spray

4 skinless boneless chicken breasts

¾ cup reduced-sugar catsup

2 tablespoons Worcestershire sauce

1 tablespoon agave nectar

1 teaspoon chili powder

DIRECTIONS

1. Preheat oven to 350 degrees.

2. Place chicken breasts in a baking pan that has been sprayed with nonstick cooking spray.

3. Bake for 20 to 25 minutes.

4. In the meantime, stir together catsup, Worcestershire sauce, agave nectar, and chili powder.

5. Remove chicken breasts from oven and coat with sauce. Return to oven and bake for 10 minutes.

YIELD: 4 servings

Bavarian Chicken Breasts

You may like your sauerkraut on a nice fattening Reuben sandwich, but try it like this instead. Sauerkraut gets its name from two German words: sauer *(sour) and* kraut *(cabbage). Historically, it was part of sailors' diets to help prevent attacks of scurvy, because of the cabbage's vitamin C content. And by the way, I have a recipe for a Reuben sandwich on page 125 . . . it's delish and won't pack on pounds!*

INGREDIENTS

1 pound sauerkraut, rinsed and drained

12 medium Brussels sprouts, stemmed and cut in half lengthwise

1 large tart green apple, peeled and coarsely shredded

¾ cup fat-free, reduced-sodium chicken broth

1 teaspoon Dijon mustard

1 teaspoon caraway seeds

1 teaspoon dried dill

Four 4-ounce boneless skinless chicken breasts

2 teaspoons mild paprika

DIRECTIONS

1. Combine the sauerkraut, Brussels sprouts, apple, broth, mustard, caraway seeds, and dill in a large, deep skillet or a Dutch oven. Bring to a boil over medium heat, stirring occasionally. Cover, reduce the heat to low, and simmer for 10 minutes.

2. Stir the sauerkraut mixture, then nestle the chicken breasts into it. Sprinkle the paprika over the chicken. Cover and continue simmering until the chicken is cooked through and the Brussels sprouts are tender, about 20 minutes.

YIELD: 4 servings

TIP: The best-tasting sauerkraut is found in plastic bags or jars in the deli case or the refrigerated meat case. Far better than the canned stuff.

Tilapia Baked in Packets

Looking to add something new to your seafood repertoire? Give tilapia a try. With recent attention focusing on the high contaminant levels of some fish, farm tilapia is a toxin-free and environmentally friendly alternative. Tilapia is a freshwater white fish with edible skin and a mild taste. It's very low in fat: A 6-ounce serving contains less than 3 grams. And, because it is digested quickly, it is a great whole-food protein source to eat before or after workouts.

INGREDIENTS

Four 16-inch sheets aluminum foil

Four 16-inch sheets parchment paper

Four 4-ounce skinless tilapia fillets

2 medium red bell peppers, stemmed, seeded, and chopped

1 pound broccoli florets

2 tablespoons minced chives

2 tablespoons minced basil leaves

1 large lemon, quartered

½ teaspoon salt

DIRECTIONS

1. Position a rack in the center of the oven and preheat to 450°F.

2. Lay the sheets of foil on your work surface; lay the sheets of parchment paper on top of the foil. Lay a tilapia fillet in the middle of each piece of parchment paper. Divide the bell peppers, broccoli florets, and herbs evenly among the servings. Squeeze lemon juice over each and sprinkle with salt. Seal the packets, crimping the seams on each side. Set them on a large baking sheet.

3. Bake for 15 minutes. Remove the baking sheet from the oven and let stand at room temperature for 5 minutes. To serve, transfer each packet to a plate and let each diner open their own—or open the packets and transfer the contents to individual bowls.

YIELD: **4 servings**

(continued on next page)

Tilapia Baked in Packets (*cont.*)

TIPS: Parchment paper is found next to aluminum foil in the supermarket. We don't recommend cooking acidic foods directly on aluminum foil. Packets are hot. Make sure you open carefully so that the escaping steam doesn't burn you.

Any thin, white-fleshed fish fillet will work: snapper, sea bass, and so on. However, the fillets must be skinned. With the skin, the fish can curl up as it cooks.

Blackened Catfish

My love affair with Cajun cooking is too hot to cool down. You'll love this blackened catfish. It's as delicious a hunk of seafood you'll ever taste. Plus, it's a healthy way to prepare the fish. Red pepper, asparagus and sugar snap peas add vitamins and phytonutrients. The flavor and tender, firm texture of catfish is an excellent source of healthy, natural protein.

INGREDIENTS

Four 4-ounce skinless catfish fillets

2 tablespoons sugar-free Cajun spice blend, grill rub, or seasoning mix

1¼ pounds cabbage, halved, cored, and coarsely shredded

1 large carrot, coarsely shredded

½ cup fat-free sour cream

1 tablespoon apple-cider vinegar

DIRECTIONS

1. Position the rack 4 to 6 inches from the broiler element; preheat.

2. Rub each catfish fillet with 1 teaspoon Cajun spice blend. Set on a rimmed baking sheet or on the broiler pan; broil 8 minutes, turning once, until deeply browned and cooked through.

3. Meanwhile, combine the cabbage, carrot, sour cream, vinegar, and the remaining 2 teaspoons Cajun spice blend in a large bowl.

4. Divide the slaw evenly among 4 plates; transfer 1 fillet onto each pile of slaw.

YIELD: 4 servings

TIP: To save time, use 5 cups bagged cole-slaw mix instead of the cabbage and carrot. Use ½ cup Walden Farms calorie-free cole-slaw dressing instead of the sour cream and vinegar. Do add the remaining Cajun spice blend to the bottled dressing to gussy it up.

Oven-Roasted Cauliflower and Broccoli

Fill up on fruits and veggies! Cruciferous vegetables, such as broccoli, cauliflower, and cabbage provide some defense against cancer. Broccoli was one of the first vegetables hailed for its anticancer properties, and it's still considered among the most potent. All three of these powerhouses contain sulforaphane, a substance that defuses potential carcinogens.

INGREDIENTS

2 pounds broccoli florets

1½ pounds cauliflower florets

4 medium garlic cloves, quartered

1 tablespoon olive oil

½ teaspoon red-pepper flakes

½ teaspoon salt

1 tablespoon balsamic vinegar

DIRECTIONS

Position a rack in the center of the oven and preheat to 400°F. Mix the broccoli, cauliflower, garlic, olive oil, red-pepper flakes, and salt in a large roasting pan or the broiler pan. Roast, stirring and tossing occasionally, until the vegetables are crisp-tender and a little browned, about 20 minutes. Remove from the oven, sprinkle with vinegar while still in hot pan, and toss well.

YIELD: 4 servings

Spicy Green Beans

Green beans are always good on their own . . . but spike them with garlic, pepper flakes, and ginger dressing, and they're great! This dish goes well with just about any entrée.

INGREDIENTS

2 teaspoons olive oil

3 medium garlic cloves, minced

½ teaspoon red-pepper flakes

1 pound green beans, stemmed

2 tablespoons low-fat, low-carb, sugar-free sesame-ginger dressing, such as Walden Farms Sesame Ginger Dressing

DIRECTIONS

1. Heat the oil in a skillet or a wok over medium-high heat. Add the garlic and red-pepper flakes; cook for 1 minute.

2. Add the green beans; toss and stir over the heat until the green beans are a little wilted, with dark brown spots, about 4 minutes. Pour in the dressing; stir for 10 seconds until green beans are coated and glazed.

YIELD: 4 servings

> **TIP:** Run the vent over your stove or open a window. The volatile oils in the red-pepper flakes can be intense. Use fat, standard green beans, not haricots verts.

Balsamic Artichokes

One of the world's oldest medicinal plants, the artichoke is loaded with powerful antioxidants that promote health and assist in liver repair. I love pulling off those succulent leaves, dipping them in low-fat salad dressing, and scraping the flesh from the leaf with my teeth. The closer you get to the "heart" of the artichoke, the more tender the leaves are. Pull off the prickly pinkish parts and scrape the silk off the heart. The heart is the most delicious part; it takes work to get there, but it's definitely worth the effort.

INGREDIENTS
> 4 fresh artichokes
> ¼ cup balsamic vinegar
> Fat-free salad dressing

DIRECTIONS

1. In a large sauce pan, bring 3 to 4 quarts of water to a boil and add balsamic vinegar. Add artichokes, cover, and cook for approximately 1 hour over medium heat, or until artichokes are tender, including the stem.

2. Let cool. Serve with fat-free salad dressing.

YIELD: 4 servings.

Green Tea–Spiked Applesauce

Did you know that apples help prevent weight gain and even aid weight loss? It's true. They contain pectin, *a substance that delays stomach emptying, keeping you full longer. Pectin also lowers cholesterol almost as effectively as drugs do.*

INGREDIENTS

4 medium tart green apples, preferably Granny Smiths, peeled, cored, and chopped

⅔ cup strong, brewed green tea

2 teaspoons Truvia

4-inch cinnamon stick

DIRECTIONS

Combine all the ingredients in a medium saucepan and bring to a bubble over medium heat. Cover, reduce heat to low, and cook, stirring occasionally, until the apples are very tender, about 30 minutes. Discard the cinnamon stick. Mash into a thick purée with the back of a wooden spoon.

YIELD: 4 servings

> **TIP:** The applesauce can be served warm or cold. Leftovers can be stored in a covered container for up to 3 days. Even better, store in one-serving ramekins or containers.

Berry Frozen Yogurt

Yes, you get to eat ice cream on the 17 Day Diet, and homemade, too. This frozen yogurt is every bit as delectable as that which you'd find in a yogurt shop.

INGREDIENTS

3 cups mixed berries, preferably 1 cup blackberries, 1 cup raspberries, and 1 cup blueberries

1 cup low-fat plain Greek yogurt

1½ tablespoons Truvia

1 teaspoon lemon juice

⅛ teaspoon salt

DIRECTIONS

1. Place all the ingredients in a blender or food processor. Cover and process until smooth, turning off the machine and scraping down the inside of the container once or twice. Refrigerate for at least 1 hour or up to 1 day.

2. Freeze in an ice-cream machine according to the manufacturer's instructions.

YIELD: 4 servings

TIP: Use frozen mixed berries. Thaw and use them with their juices.

Chocolaty Frozen Yogurt

If you love chocolate ice cream, you'll love this recipe. It will definitely keep you from plunging headlong into a gallon of your favorite chocolate ice cream.

INGREDIENTS

12 ounces Greek 2% yogurt

1 tablespoons low-fat buttermilk

1 tablespoons agave nectar

2 teaspoons unsweetened cocoa

¼ cup Nestle's Quik sugar-free hot cocoa mix

½ teaspoon instant espresso powder

½ teaspoon vanilla extract

DIRECTIONS

1. Combine all ingredients. Mix well using a whisk.

2. Refrigerate for a few hours until mixture very cold.

3. Freeze in an ice-cream machine according to manufacturer's instructions.

YIELD: 2 servings

Spiced Plum Soup

Soup's on in the form of a sweet dessert. Soup is filling, so save room for this!

INGREDIENTS

1 pound red or black plums, pitted and coarsely chopped
1½ cups water
1½ tablespoons Truvia
1½ teaspoons ground cinnamon
¼ teaspoon ground cloves
½ cup plain, low-fat, Greek yogurt
Chopped mint leaves, optional

DIRECTIONS

1. Combine the plums, water, Truvia, cinnamon, and cloves in a medium saucepan. Bring to a simmer over medium heat, stirring occasionally. Cover, reduce heat to low, and simmer very slowly until the plums have softened, about 15 minutes, stirring occasionally.

2. Cool for 10 minutes. Transfer the entire contents of the saucepan to a large blender or food processor. Add the yogurt, cover, and process until smooth. Chill for at least 1 hour before serving. Garnish with chopped mint leaves, if desired.

YIELD: 4 servings

> **TIP:** If you like a kick in your sweet desserts, the soup is nice with ⅛ teaspoon cayenne added with the cinnamon and cloves. Store the soup, covered, in the fridge for up to 4 days.

17 Sample Cycle 1 Menus

Here are examples of how you can create your daily menu using the Accelerate Cycle recipes.

Day 1

Breakfast

☐ 1 serving *Snappy Eggs*

☐ ½ grapefruit or other fresh fruit

☐ 1 cup green tea

Lunch

☐ 1 serving *California Tuna Salad*

☐ 1 cup green tea

Dinner

☐ 1 serving *Tandoori Chicken Breasts*

☐ 1 cup green tea

Snack

☐ 6 ounces nonfat yogurt mixed with 1 or 2 tablespoons sugar-free jam

☐ 1 serving Cycle 1 fruit

Day 2

Breakfast

☐ 1 serving *Peach Melba Smoothie*

☐ 1 cup green tea

Lunch

☐ 1 serving *Super Salad*

☐ 1 cup green tea

Dinner

☐ 1 serving *Blackened Catfish* with liberal amounts of any Cycle 1 vegetables, steamed or raw

☐ 1 cup green tea

Snack

☐ 6 ounces sugar-free fruit-flavored yogurt, or 1 cup plain low-fat yogurt, sweetened with Truvia or a tablespoon of sugar-free fruit jam

☐ 1 serving fruit

Day 3

Breakfast

- ☐ 1 serving *Mushroom Spinach Frittata*
- ☐ ½ grapefruit or other fresh fruit in season
- ☐ 1 cup green tea

Lunch

- ☐ 1 large bowl *Chicken-Vegetable Soup*
- ☐ 1 cup green tea

Dinner

- ☐ Plenty of roasted turkey breast or turkey tenderloin, steamed carrots, and steamed asparagus.
- ☐ 1 cup green tea

Snack

- ☐ 6 ounces plain nonfat yogurt, sweetened with Truvia or a tablespoon of sugar-free fruit jam
- ☐ *Kefir Smoothie*

Day 4

Breakfast

☐ *Kefir Smoothie*

☐ 1 cup green tea

Lunch

☐ 1 serving *Turkey Picadillo Lettuce Wraps*

Dinner

☐ 1 serving *No-Fuss Eggplant Parm*

☐ 1 cup green tea

Snack

☐ 6 ounces plain nonfat yogurt with a sliced fresh peach, or other fruit in season

☐ 1 cup green tea

Day 5

Breakfast

- ☐ 2 scrambled egg whites
- ☐ ½ grapefruit or other fresh fruit in season
- ☐ 1 cup green tea

Lunch

- ☐ 1 serving *Super Salad*
- ☐ 1 cup green tea

Dinner

- ☐ 1 serving *Stir-Fried Chicken and Cucumbers*
- ☐ 1 cup green tea

Snacks

- ☐ 1 cup fresh berries
- ☐ 6 ounces plain nonfat yogurt, sweetened with Truvia or a table-spoon of sugar-free fruit jam

NOTES

Day 6

Breakfast

☐ 6 ounces nonfat yogurt, mixed with 1 cup berries, or other fruit on the list. You may sweeten with 1 packet of Truvia or a tablespoon of sugar-free fruit jam.

☐ 1 cup green tea

Lunch

☐ Grilled chicken breast with tossed salad drizzled with 1 tablespoon of olive or flaxseed oil and 2 tablespoons balsamic vinegar

☐ 1 cup green tea

Dinner

☐ 1 serving *Curried Poached Halibut*

☐ 1 cup green tea

Snacks

☐ 1 serving *Spiced Plum Soup*

☐ 2nd probiotic serving of your choice

Day 7

Breakfast

- ☐ 1 serving *Snappy Eggs*
- ☐ 1 apple or 1 cup fresh berries
- ☐ 1 cup green tea

Lunch

- ☐ 1 serving *Super Salad*
- ☐ 1 cup green tea

Dinner

- ☐ 1 serving *Bavarian Chicken Breasts*
- ☐ 1 cup green tea

Snacks

- ☐ 2nd fruit serving + 1 probiotic serving of your choice
- ☐ 2nd probiotic serving of your choice

Day 8

Breakfast

☐ 6 ounces nonfat yogurt, mixed with 1 cup berries, or other fruit on the list. You may sweeten with 1 packet of Truvia or a tablespoon of sugar-free fruit jam.

☐ 1 cup green tea

Lunch

☐ 1 serving *Lemon-Pepper Salmon Salad in Tomato Cups*

☐ 1 cup green tea

Dinner

☐ Turkey burgers (made with lean ground turkey)

☐ Steamed Cycle 1 vegetables

☐ Side salad drizzled with drizzled with 1 tablespoon olive or flax-seed oil, mixed with 2 tablespoons balsamic vinegar and seasonings

☐ 1 cup green tea

Snack

☐ 1 serving *Berry Frozen Yogurt*

Day 9

Breakfast

- ☐ 1 serving *Greek Egg Scramble*
- ☐ 1 fresh orange
- ☐ 1 cup green tea

Lunch

- ☐ 1 serving *Grilled Tuna Niçoise Salad*
- ☐ 1 cup green tea

Dinner

- ☐ Grilled chicken breast marinated in fat-free Italian dressing, then broiled or grilled
- ☐ Steamed Cycle 1 vegetables
- ☐ 1 cup green tea

Snacks

- ☐ *Peach Melba Smoothie*
- ☐ 6 ounces nonfat yogurt sweetened with Truvia or no-sugar jam

Day 10

Breakfast

☐ ½ cup Breakstone LiveActive cottage cheese

☐ 1 medium pear, sliced

☐ 1 cup green tea

Lunch

☐ 1 *Balsamic Artichoke*, served with nonfat salad dressing

☐ 1 serving *Green Tea–Spiked Applesauce*

☐ 1 cup green tea

Dinner

☐ 1 serving *Oven-Barbecued Chicken*

☐ Side salad drizzled with 1 tablespoon olive or flaxseed oil, mixed with 2 tablespoons balsamic vinegar and seasonings

☐ 1 cup green tea

Snacks

☐ 2nd probiotic serving

☐ Raw cut-up veggies

Day 11

Breakfast

- ☐ 1 serving *Yogurt Fruitshake*
- ☐ 1 cup green tea

Lunch

- ☐ 1 serving *Super Salad*
- ☐ 1 cup green tea

Dinner

- ☐ Ground turkey patties
- ☐ 1 serving *Oven-Roasted Cauliflower and Broccoli*
- ☐ 1 cup green tea

Snacks

- ☐ 1 serving *Berry Frozen Yogurt*

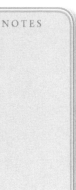

NOTES

Day 12

Breakfast

- ☐ 2 hard-boiled or poached eggs
- ☐ ½ grapefruit or other fresh fruit
- ☐ 1 cup green tea

Lunch

- ☐ Baked or grilled chicken breast
- ☐ Tomatoes, sliced or stewed
- ☐ 1 cup green tea

Dinner

- ☐ 1 serving *Tilapia Baked in Packets*
- ☐ 1 cup green tea

Snacks

- ☐ 1 serving *Kefir Smoothie*
- ☐ 1 serving *Berry Frozen Yogurt*

Day 13

Breakfast

☐ 1 serving *Peach Melba Smoothie*

☐ 1 cup green tea

Lunch

☐ 1 serving *California Tuna Salad*

☐ 1 cup green tea

Dinner

☐ Plenty of roast turkey or chicken

☐ 1 serving *Spicy Green Beans*

☐ 1 cup green tea

Snacks

☐ 2nd fruit serving

☐ 1 serving *Berry Frozen Yogurt*

Day 14

Breakfast

- ☐ 1 serving of *Mushroom Spinach Frittata*
- ☐ 1 apple or 1 cup fresh berries
- ☐ 1 cup green tea

Lunch

- ☐ 1 large bowl *Chicken-Vegetable Soup*
- ☐ 1 cup green tea

Dinner

- ☐ 1 serving *Tandoori Chicken Breasts*
- ☐ 1 cup green tea

Snacks

- ☐ 1 medium pear or other fruit
- ☐ 6 ounces nonfat yogurt sweetened with Truvia or no-sugar jam

Day 15

Breakfast

☐ ½ cup Breakstone LiveActive cottage cheese

☐ 1 medium pear, sliced

☐ 1 cup green tea

Lunch

☐ 1 serving *No-Fuss Eggplant Parm*

☐ 1 cup green tea

Dinner

☐ 1 serving *Low-Carb Primavera Delight*

☐ 1 cup green tea

Snacks

☐ 2nd fruit serving

☐ 1 serving *Berry Frozen Yogurt*

NOTES

Breakfast

☐ 1 serving *Spanish Omelet*

☐ ½ grapefruit or 1 medium orange

☐ 1 cup green tea

Lunch

☐ 1 serving *Creamy Smoked Salmon Rolls*

☐ 1 cup green tea

Dinner

☐ Plenty of roasted turkey breast or turkey tenderloin, steamed carrots, and steamed asparagus.

☐ 1 cup green tea

Snacks

☐ 1 piece fresh fruit

☐ 6 ounces nonfat yogurt sweetened with Truvia or no-sugar jam

Day 17

Breakfast

- ☐ 1 serving *Yogurt Fruitshake*
- ☐ 1 cup green tea

Lunch

- ☐ 1 serving *Super Salad*
- ☐ 1 cup green tea

Dinner

- ☐ 1 serving *Tilapia in Packets*
- ☐ 1 cup green tea

Snacks

- ☐ 1 medium apple
- ☐ 1 serving *Berry Frozen Yogurt*

RECIPES

Cycle 2—Activate

GOAL: To reset your metabolism through a strategy that involves increasing and decreasing your caloric consumption to stimulate fat-burning and to help prevent plateaus.

Dr. Mike's Power Cookie

My experience in medicine convinced me that the best approach to both snacks and meals is to present a varied diet with numerous choices, which is why I give you cookies! Yes, imagine being able to eat cookies on a diet. Well, now you can. I keep a large wide-mouthed jar full of these nutritious cookies. They are high in protein, very satisfying, and have sweet-tooth appeal. Include these in your plan, and you'll feel and look like one smart cookie.

INGREDIENTS

⅓ cup unsweetened applesauce

2 tablespoons almond paste

1 tablespoon flaxseed oil

10 packets of Truvia

¼ cup agave nectar

1 large egg

½ teaspoon vanilla

¾ cup whole-wheat flour

½ teaspoon baking soda

1 teaspoon cinnamon

½ teaspoon salt

¼ teaspoon black pepper

½ cup vanilla whey powder

2 cups oats

1 cup dried cherries

½ cup sliced almonds

Nonstick cooking spray

DIRECTIONS

1. Heat oven to 350 degrees. Beat together applesauce, almond paste, flaxseed oil, Truvia, and agave nectar. Beat in egg and vanilla. Mix well. Add flour, baking soda, cinnamon, salt, pepper, and whey powder. Beat thoroughly. Stir in oats, cherries, and almonds. Mix well.

(continued on next page)

Dr. Mike's Power Cookie (*cont.*)

2. Drop the batter by large tablespoons onto a cookie sheet that has been sprayed with nonstick cooking spray. Divide dough into 18 balls. Flatten cookies with the back of a spoon. Bake 16 to 18 minutes or until soft and brown. Remove from oven. Cool and store in a covered container.

YIELD: 18 cookies

> **TIP:** Each cookie supplies 128 calories and can be enjoyed on the Activate, Achieve, and Arrive cycles for breakfast or as a snack. Each cookie counts as 1 protein and 1 natural starch.

Eggs, Lox, and Onions

Call me a little crazy, but I dig fish first thing in the morning, if it's lox, that is. There's just nothing better than good smoked salmon. Normally, lox is served with bagels, smeared with cream cheese. Here it's paired with eggs, and what a great match it is. You won't miss your bagel.

INGREDIENTS

2 teaspoons olive oil

1 small yellow onion, chopped fine

2 large eggs

2 large egg whites

4 ounces lox or smoked salmon, chopped

½ teaspoon black pepper

DIRECTIONS

1. Heat the oil in a large nonstick skillet over medium heat. Add the onion. Cook, stirring often, until softened and lightly browned, about 6 minutes.

2. Whisk the eggs and egg whites in a large bowl until well blended. Pour into the skillet; reduce the heat to low. Stir until curds begin to form. Add the salmon and pepper; continue stirring until the eggs are set, about 1 minute.

YIELD: 2 servings (can be doubled)

> **TIP:** You can substitute smoked trout or smoked mackerel for salmon in this recipe.

Weekend Morning Grits Casserole

I'm particularly proud of this dish, and my vegetarian friends love it. The casserole has everything you need for a good hearty breakfast: whole grains, protein, veggies, and fruit.

INGREDIENTS

Nonstick cooking spray

½ cup quick-cooking grits

6 ounces soy sausage, crumbled, or sausage-flavored textured soy protein

4 medium scallions, minced

1 tablespoon Worcestershire sauce

1 tablespoon minced fresh oregano leaves or 1 teaspoon dried oregano

¼ teaspoon garlic powder

1 tart green apple, peeled and coarsely grated

4 ounces grated fat-free Cheddar or Parmesan cheese

1 large egg

1 large egg white

DIRECTIONS

1. Bring 2 cups water to a boil in a large saucepan over high heat. Stir in the grits, reduce the heat, and simmer, stirring almost constantly, until thick, about 4 minutes.

2. Remove the pan from the heat. Stir in the sausage, scallions, Worcestershire sauce, oregano, and garlic powder. Set aside for 10 minutes.

3. Meanwhile, position a rack in the center of the oven; preheat to 375°F. Lightly spray the inside of an 8-inch square baking pan with nonstick cooking spray.

4. Stir in the apple and cheese. Pour and spread this mixture into the prepared baking pan.

5. Bake until puffed, brown, and set, about 25 minutes. Cool for 5 minutes before cutting into squares.

YIELD: 4 servings

Super Strawberry Smoothie

If you're not into smoothies for breakfast, we need to talk. These blended drinks are the quickest breakfasts you can imagine, as well as being a super-healthy way to start the day. I like making mine with yogurt. In addition to being a good source of protein and calcium, its low levels of lactose are easy for everyone to tolerate. And remember, probiotics like yogurt and kefir are fat-burners par excellence.

INGREDIENTS

1 cup frozen strawberries, partially thawed

6-ounces sugar-free low-fat strawberry yogurt

¼ cup plain, low-fat kefir

1 tablespoon oat bran

¼ teaspoon grated nutmeg

2 ice cubes

DIRECTIONS

Place all the ingredients in a blender. Cover and blend until smooth, pulsing occasionally to make sure everything is well blended, and scraping down the inside of the container once or twice after turning the blender off.

YIELD: 1 serving

TIP: If the berries are really hard, it helps to rock the blender a bit.

Italian Shrimp and White Bean Salad

When you see shrimp as an ingredient in many recipes, it's usually a good sign, because the recipes are probably low in calories and high in fat-burning protein, Another ingredient is white beans, which provide filling, satisfying fiber. This shrimp salad balances taste, texture, and nutrition to great effect. So there you have it: savory, smooth, and tangy. And healthy. This is an easy salad to make, too.

INGREDIENTS
½ pound medium shrimp, peeled and deveined
1 can (15 ounces) white beans, drained and rinsed
3 medium celery stalks, minced
½ small red onion, minced
¼ cup low-fat, no-sugar, creamy Italian dressing

DIRECTIONS
1. Bring a large saucepan of water to a boil. Add the shrimp. Cook until pink and firm, about 3 minutes. Drain in a colander. Rinse with cool tap water to stop the cooking. Drain thoroughly by shaking the colander.

2. Chop the shrimp on a cutting board, then place in a serving bowl. Add the beans, celery, onion, and dressing; stir well.

YIELD: 2 servings (can be doubled)

> **TIP:** To save time, use cooked, peeled, and deveined cocktail shrimp. You can stir everything together in minutes.

Crab Tabouleh

Tabouleh is a traditional Middle Eastern salad featuring vegetables and bulgur wheat. This recipe adds crab, which enhances the other ingredients remarkably well.

INGREDIENTS

½ cup quick-cooking bulgur

6 ounces crabmeat, picked over for bits of shell and cartilage

1 cup canned chickpeas, drained and rinsed

½ cup frozen corn, thawed

2 medium scallions, sliced thin

1 roasted red pepper, chopped

¼ cup low-fat, no-sugar balsamic vinaigrette

DIRECTIONS

1. Bring 2 cups water to a boil in a small saucepan over high heat.

2. Place the bulgur in a large, heat-safe mixing bowl. Pour the boiling water over the bulgur; set aside until the water has been absorbed, about 20 minutes.

3. Stir in the crabmeat, chickpeas, corn, scallions, red pepper, and vinaigrette.

YIELD: 2 servings (can be doubled)

> **TIP:** Pasteurized crabmeat is available in cans, usually in the refrigerator case near the fish counter. It's tastier than the shelf-stable, tinned stuff. However, pasteurized crabmeat does need to be put on a plate or cutting board and picked over in case there are any fragments of bone or shell. By the way, no need to buy the more expensive jumbo lump or lump crabmeat for this, just regular crabmeat.

Warm Curried Quinoa Salad

Quinoa is lower in carbohydrates than most grains and is an excellent source of protein. It's highly nutritious, very tasty, easy to prepare, and great if you're gluten intolerant. Featuring roasted red peppers, onions, garlic, and ginger, and more in a taste-bud–bursting dressing, this salad is fantastic.

INGREDIENTS

½ cup beige or red quinoa

Nonstick cooking spray

1 small yellow onion, chopped

1 tablespoon peeled, minced fresh ginger or prepared minced ginger

1 medium garlic clove, minced, or 1 teaspoon prepared minced garlic

1 tablespoon curry powder

¼ teaspoon salt

1 bag (8 ounces) cole-slaw mix

1½ tablespoons apple-cider vinegar

1 medium sweet apple, like Gala or Fuji, peeled and coarsely shredded

3 tablespoons low-fat, no-sugar bottled ranch dressing

DIRECTIONS

1. Bring 1 cup water to a boil in a medium saucepan over high heat. Stir in the quinoa. Reduce the heat to low; cook until the water has been absorbed and the quinoa is tender, about 12 minutes.

2. Spray a large nonstick skillet with nonstick cooking spray. Set over medium heat for 1 minute, then add the onion, ginger, and garlic. Cook, stirring often, until softened, about 3 minutes. Stir in the curry powder and salt; cook until fragrant, about 20 seconds.

3. Add the slaw mix and vinegar. Scrape up any browned bits on the skillet's bottom as the vinegar comes to a boil. Cover, reduce the heat to low, and cook until the cabbage is tender, about 10 minutes.

4. Remove the skillet from the heat. Stir in the apple, cooked quinoa, and dressing.

YIELD: 2 servings

> **TIP:** For an on-the-go lunch, make ahead and warm in the microwave.
> Some quinoa has a bitter chemical compound—*saponin*—still on the seeds. Most have been washed to remove this compound. However, if you buy quinoa in bulk or inexpensive packaging in international markets, you probably should rinse the quinoa in a colander before cooking to remove this compound.

Smoked Turkey and Lentil Salad

Diets are synonymous with salads. Instead of just tossing together some lettuce, celery, tomato, and a splatter of dressing, why not try new flavor combinations? You can turn a salad into something exceptional with just a few interesting ingredients, like lentils, a staple of vegetarians and the popular Mediterranean diet. I love lentils in any form; they're rich in protein, vitamin B, and iron, and taste great with smoked turkey and spices here.

INGREDIENTS

¾ cup green lentils

6 ounces deli-type smoked turkey, diced

3 medium celery stalks, minced

1 large carrot, coarsely grated

¼ cup low-fat, no-sugar, bottled creamy Italian vinaigrette

2 teaspoons fresh thyme leaves or ½ teaspoon dried thyme

½ teaspoon ground black pepper

DIRECTIONS

1. Fill a large saucepan about two-thirds full with water; bring to a boil over high heat. Add the lentils; reduce the heat to low. Simmer until tender, about 15 minutes. Drain the lentils in a colander. Rinse with cool tap water to stop the cooking. Drain thoroughly, shaking the colander.

2. Pour the lentils into a large bowl. Stir in the turkey, celery, carrot, dressing, thyme, and pepper.

YIELD: 2 servings

Falafel Salad

Falafel is made from chick peas, bulgur wheat, and spices. It is high in fiber and protein, and has no cholesterol. Added to a salad, it may make the perfect vegetarian meal.

INGREDIENTS

½ cup quick-cooking bulgur
1 cup canned chickpeas, drained and rinsed
¼ cup parsley leaves
2 medium scallions, sliced thin
1 medium garlic clove, peeled
1 large egg white
1 teaspoon baking powder
1 teaspoon ground cumin
½ teaspoon cinnamon
½ teaspoon salt
½ teaspoon black pepper
1 tablespoon olive oil
1 bag (9 ounces) Romaine salad mix
1 large tomato, chopped
1 medium cucumber, peeled and chopped
½ cup low-fat, sugar-free, bottled ranch dressing

DIRECTIONS

1. Bring 1 cup water to a boil over high heat in a small saucepan. Put the bulgur in a large, heat-safe bowl. Pour the boiling water over the bulgur. Set aside until the water has been absorbed, about 30 minutes.

2. Scrape the bulgur into a large food processor fitted with a chopping blade. Add the chickpeas, parsley, scallions, garlic, egg white, baking powder, cumin, cinnamon, salt, and pepper. Cover and blend until the mixture becomes a grainy paste, scraping down

(continued on next page)

Falafel Salad (*cont.*)

the inside of the canister once or twice after shutting the machine off. Scrape down and remove the blade from the food processor.

3. Heat the oil in a large nonstick skillet over medium heat. With wet hands, pat the paste into four patties, slipping them one by one into the skillet. Cook until brown and fairly dry on one side, about 4 minutes. Turn the patties and continue cooking until brown and set, about 4 more minutes. Transfer to a cutting board.

4. Mix the salad greens, tomato, cucumber, and dressing in a large bowl. Divide among four plates. Top with a falafel patty.

YIELD: 4 servings

> **TIP:** For an on-the-go lunch, keep the salad dressing separate from the greens until you're ready to eat. The falafel patties freeze well. Once thoroughly cooled, wrap in plastic and store in the freezer for up to 3 months. Warm in a dry skillet over medium heat for a few minutes, turning once; or on a baking sheet in a preheated 350°F oven for 10 minutes.

Cantonese Stir-Fried Shrimp

I thought I'd just go ahead and get the preachy eat-more-veggies sermon out of the way now. You'll certainly do that with this recipe. It's very similar to the shrimp-with-snow-peas dish you find in many Cantonese restaurants. But there are even more veggies in this version.

INGREDIENTS

Nonstick cooking spray

2 medium scallions, minced

1 tablespoon minced peeled fresh ginger or prepared minced ginger

1 minced medium garlic clove or 1 teaspoon prepared minced garlic

6 ounces thinly sliced cremini or white button mushrooms

1 pound medium shrimp, peeled and deveined

6 ounces snow peas, trimmed

1 can (14 ounces) baby corn, drained and rinsed

2 tablespoons fat-free, low-sodium chicken broth

1 tablespoon light soy sauce

1 tablespoon oyster sauce, optional

DIRECTIONS

1. Spray a large wok, preferably nonstick, with nonstick cooking spray. Set it over high heat just until smoking, about 3 minutes. Add the scallions, ginger, and garlic. Toss and stir over the heat until aromatic, about 30 seconds.

2. Add the mushrooms; stir-fry for 1 minute. Add the shrimp and continue tossing and stirring over the heat for 1 minute.

3. Add the snow peas and corn. Stir-fry for 1 minute. Pour in the broth; keep stir-frying until the wok is almost dry, about another minute. Finally, add the soy sauce and the oyster sauce, if using. Toss a few times before serving.

YIELD: 4 servings

(continued on next page)

Cantonese Stir-Fried Shrimp (*cont.*)

TIPS: Have bags of frozen shrimp on hand in Cycle 2. To thaw more quickly, place in a bowl, cover with water, and let stand for 10 minutes, changing the water once. Oyster sauce is an option here because it's so very Cantonese. It's available in the Asian aisle of most supermarkets.

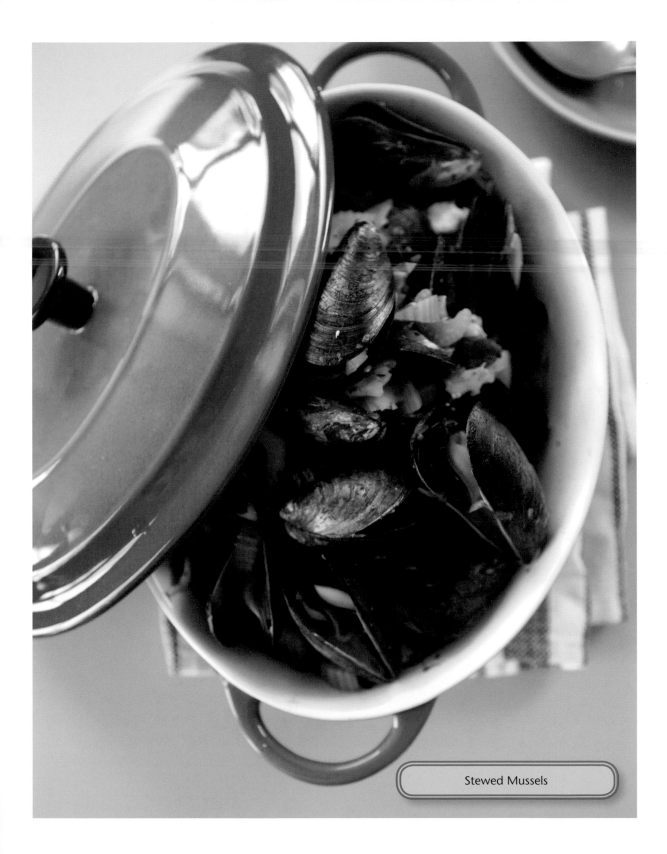

Stewed Mussels

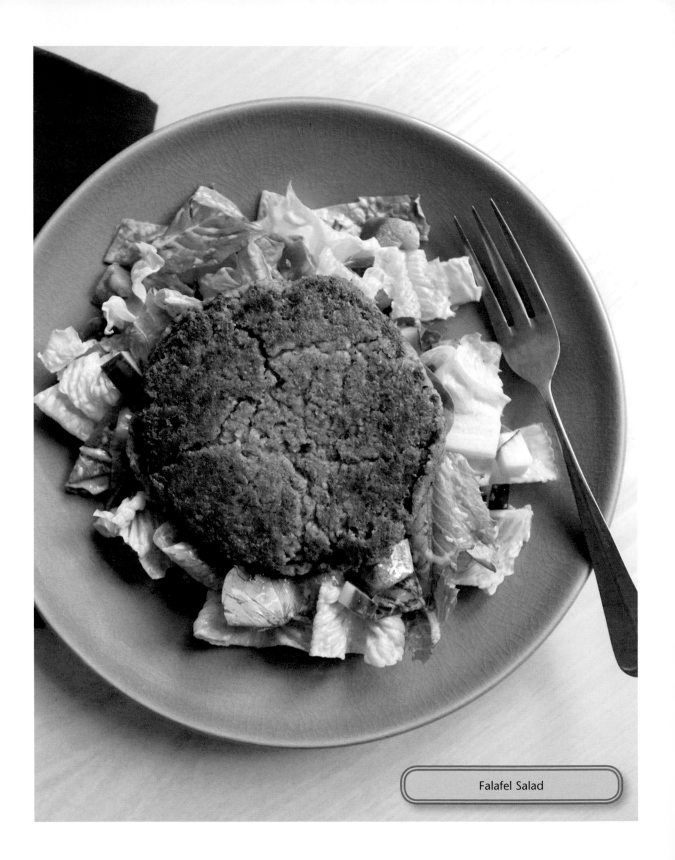

Falafel Salad

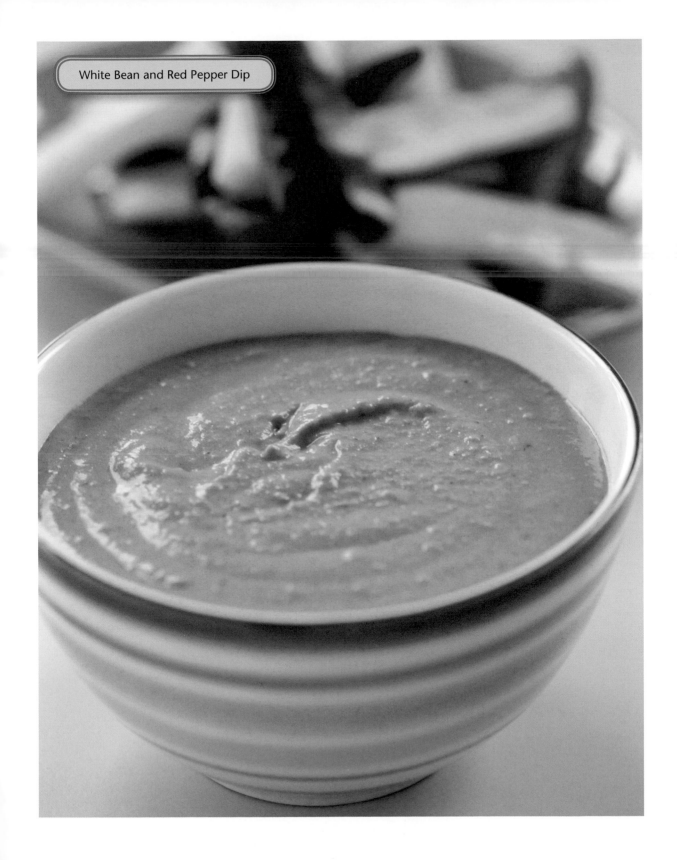

White Bean and Red Pepper Dip

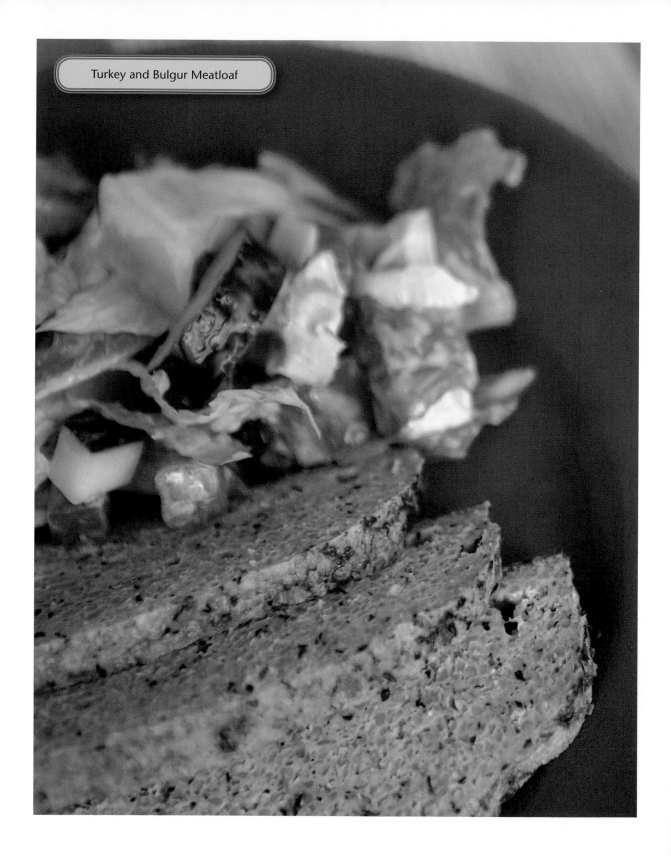

Turkey and Bulgur Meatloaf

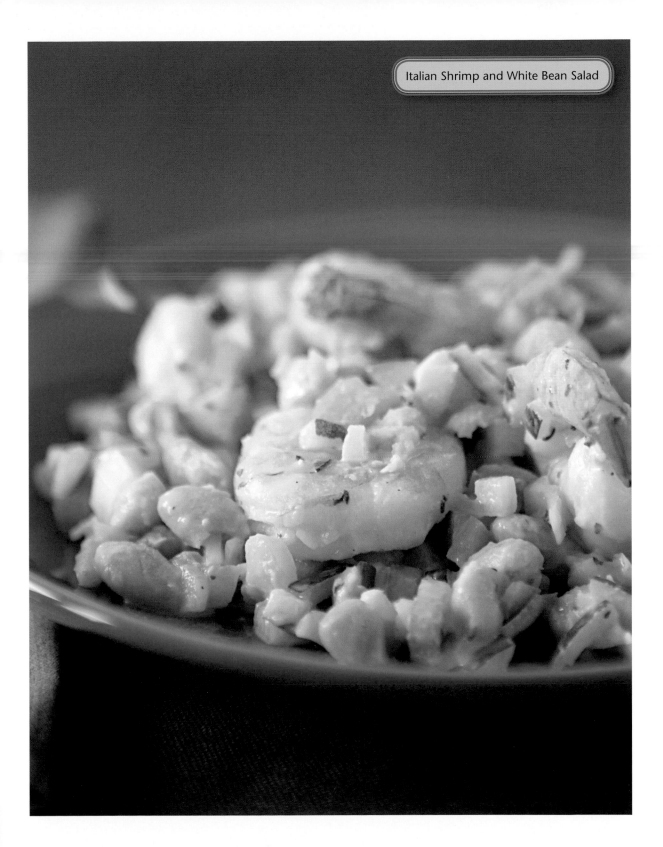

Italian Shrimp and White Bean Salad

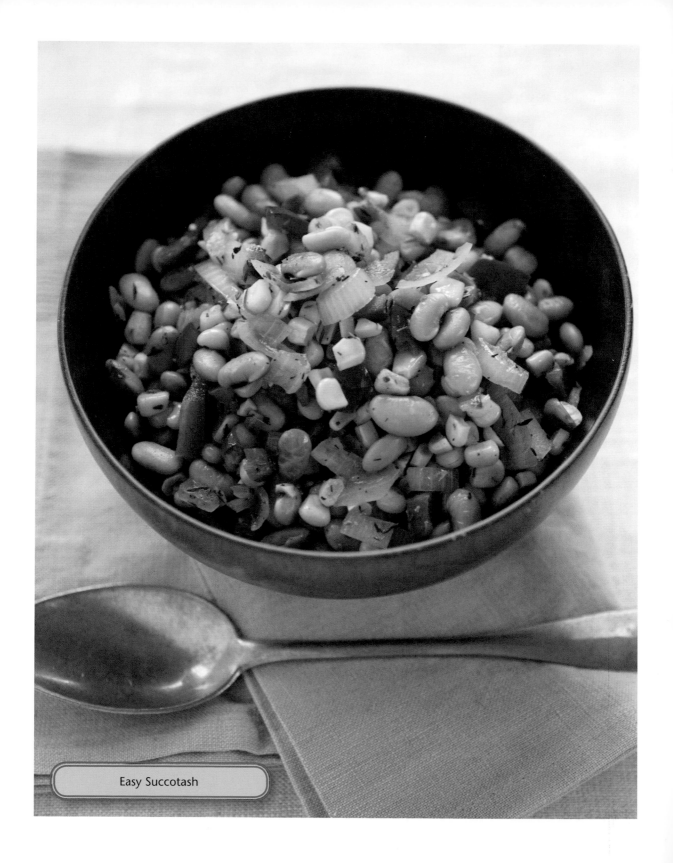

Easy Succotash

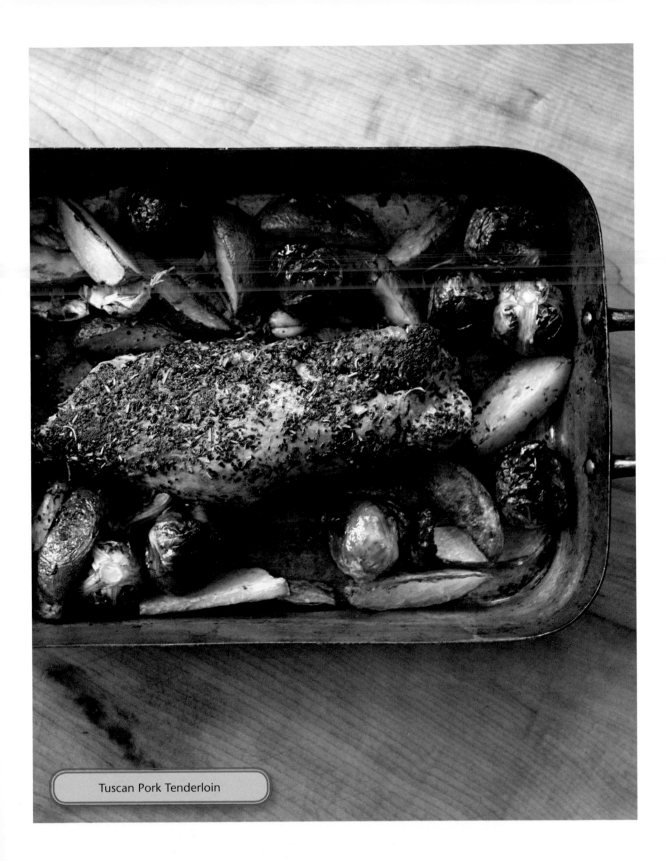

Tuscan Pork Tenderloin

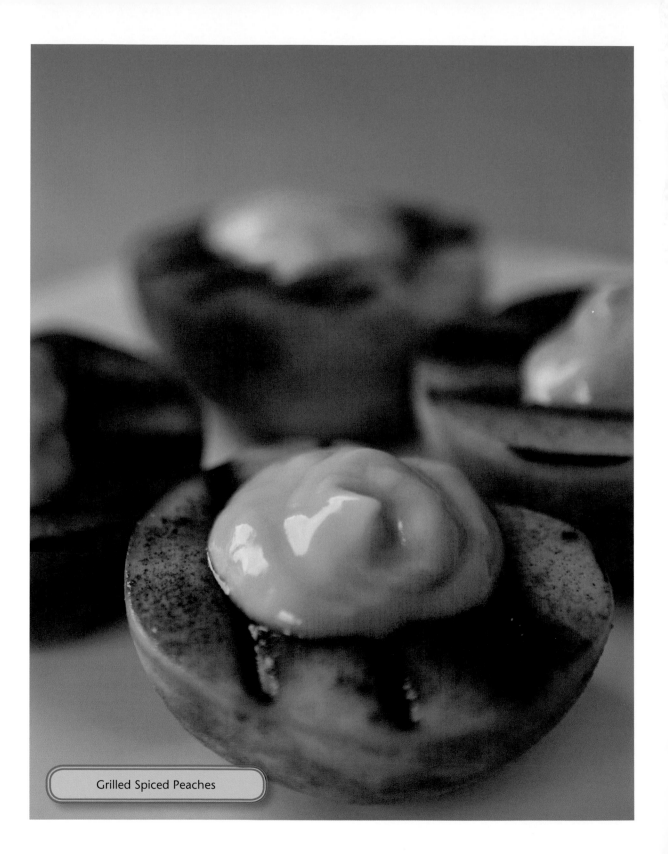

Grilled Spiced Peaches

Roasted Shrimp and Broccoli

No time to cook dinner? Well, if you can fit in just 12 minutes, here's the dinner for you. It's a superquick one-pot meal that you can dish up in no time.

INGREDIENTS

- 1½ pounds frozen broccoli florets, thawed
- 1 pound (about 30) peeled and deveined medium shrimp
- 1 tablespoon olive oil
- 1 tablespoon lemon juice
- 2 minced medium garlic cloves or 2 teaspoons prepared minced garlic
- 1 teaspoon finely grated lemon zest
- ½ teaspoon red-pepper flakes
- ½ teaspoon salt

DIRECTIONS

1. Position the rack in the center of the oven; preheat the oven to 425°F.
2. Mix all the ingredients in a large roasting pan or the broiler pan. Bake until the shrimp are pink and firm, about 12 minutes, tossing once or twice.

YIELD: 4 servings

TIP: You can find already peeled and deveined shrimp at almost every supermarket. Just don't use cooked cocktail shrimp.

Stewed Mussels

Many people are shy of mussels, but I love them no matter how they're prepared. Cooked mussels, grilled mussels, fried mussels, and now stewed mussels: A meal of mussels is the meal for me. But no mussel recipe has ever tasted so good to me as this one. Mussels are low in fat, high in omega 3s, and packed with high levels of daily requirements for zinc, vitamin C, and iron.

INGREDIENTS

1 medium yellow onion, chopped

4 medium celery stalks, minced

1 can (28 ounces) reduced-sodium diced tomatoes

1 can (14 ounces) artichoke-heart quarters packed in water, drained and rinsed

2 tablespoons minced fresh oregano leaves or 2 teaspoons dried oregano

2 tablespoons fresh thyme leaves or 2 teaspoons dried thyme

½ teaspoon red-pepper flakes, optional

4 pounds mussels, cleaned and debearded

DIRECTIONS

1. Combine the onion, celery, tomatoes, artichokes, oregano, thyme, and red-pepper flakes, if using, in a very large pot or Dutch oven. Bring to a boil over high heat. Reduce the heat to low, cover, and simmer slowly for 10 minutes.

2. Stir in the mussels. Raise the heat to medium, cover, and continue cooking until the mussels open, about 12 minutes. Pour the contents of the pot into a large serving bowl. Discard any mussels that do not open.

YIELD: 4 servings

TIPS: Ask for a small bag of ice from the supermarket or fishmonger to keep mussels cool, particularly on a warm day. Place them in a large bowl and refrigerate. To debeard mussels, pull the wiry threads from their shells along the seam until they snap free. Rinse to remove any sand. Do not cook any mussels that are open and refuse to shut when tapped. Cook mussels on the same day you buy them.

Easy Chicken Posole

You'll go crazy over this chicken posole, a hearty stew with a Southwestern attitude, based on green chili peppers, cumin, and garlic. This dish, which calls for canned hominy, takes a fraction of the time needed for regular posole.

INGREDIENTS

Nonstick cooking spray

1 medium yellow onion, chopped

1 medium red bell pepper, stemmed, cored, and chopped

1 medium garlic clove, minced, or 1 teaspoon prepared minced garlic

1 pound boneless skinless chicken breasts, cut into 1-inch pieces

2 cans (15 ounces) hominy, drained and rinsed

1 can (4 ounces) chopped green chilies, mild or hot

2 teaspoons dried oregano

1 teaspoon ground cumin

1½ cups fat-free, low-sodium chicken broth

¼ cup fat-free sour cream, optional

¼ cup minced cilantro leaves

Lime wedges, optional

DIRECTIONS

1. Spray a large saucepan with nonstick cooking spray; set the pan over medium heat for 1 minute. Add the onion, bell pepper, and garlic; cook, stirring often, until softened, about 3 minutes.

2. Stir in the chicken breasts. Continue cooking, stirring often, until the chicken loses its raw, pink color, about 5 minutes.

3. Add the hominy, chilies, oregano, and cumin; stir for 1 minute. Pour in the broth; raise the heat to high and stir occasionally as the mixture comes to a boil. Cover, reduce the heat to low, and simmer for 20 minutes. Ladle into serving bowls; top each with 1 tablespoon sour cream, if using, and 1 tablespoon minced cilantro. Serve with lime wedges on the side to squeeze into the stew, if using.

YIELD: 4 servings

TIP: To save time, you can use frozen chopped onions in place of a chopped onion. One medium yellow onion = 1 cup frozen chopped onion. No need to thaw frozen chopped onions. Use them straight from the freezer.

Turkey and Bulgur Meatloaf

When it's cold, snowy, or rainy outside, what else is there to do but snuggle up to a plate of meatloaf? The problem is that traditional meatloaf can be loaded with fat and calories, a dish that can latch right on to your hips and thighs. This recipe reduces all the bad stuff without being a traitor to tradition. Using ground turkey and bulgur instead of high-carb bread crumbs helps you keep a careful watch over your diet. Dig in, and you'll get a hefty dose of nutrition. This no-fuss recipe will have your loved ones saying, "Make that again, please!"

INGREDIENTS

½ cup quick-cooking bulgur
Nonstick cooking spray
1 pound lean ground turkey
1 large egg white
1 tablespoon Dijon mustard
1½ teaspoons salt-free Italian spice or seasoning blend
½ teaspoon salt
½ teaspoon ground black pepper

DIRECTIONS

1. Bring ¾ cup water to a boil in a small saucepan over high heat. Meanwhile, place the bulgur in a large blender; cover and blend until finely ground, about 1 minute. Pour the ground bulgur into the boiling water, cover, and set aside off the heat until cool, about 30 minutes.

2. Position the rack in the center of the oven and preheat the oven to 350°F. Spray a 9- x 13-inch baking dish lightly with nonstick cooking spray.

3. Pour the bulgur into a large bowl; fluff with a fork. Mix in the ground turkey, egg white, mustard, spice blend, salt, and pepper. Form the mixture into an oval mound; set on a baking pan.

4. Bake until browned and cooked through, about 50 minutes. Cool for 5 minutes before slicing.

YIELD: 4 servings

> **TIP:** Want to be fancy? Smear the top of the unbaked meatloaf with 2 teaspoons Dijon mustard, sugar-free barbecue sauce, Worcestershire sauce, or sugar-free catsup.

Fast and Easy Chili

If you take a look under the hood of many chili recipes, you'll often find a lot of fattening ingredients, like fatty cuts of meat or too much oil. That said, let's design the perfect chili recipe. It has to be low-low fat and high in protein. It should be loaded with vitamins and minerals and have gobs of complex carbohydrates and fiber. And . . . and . . . oh, yeah. It should taste great. Know what we just designed? Fast and Easy Chili.

INGREDIENTS

Nonstick cooking spray

1 pound lean ground beef

1 can (15 ounces) kidney beans, drained and rinsed

2 cups prepared mild or medium salsa

1 cup frozen corn kernels

2 tablespoons chili powder

2 teaspoons lime juice

1 teaspoon ground cumin

¼ cup fat-free sour cream, optional

DIRECTIONS

1. Spray a large saucepan with nonstick cooking spray. Set over medium heat, then crumble in the ground beef. Cook, stirring often, until lightly browned, about 4 minutes.

2. Stir in the beans, salsa sauce, corn, chili powder, lime juice, and cumin. Bring to a full simmer. Cover, reduce the heat to low, and cook for 15 minutes, stirring occasionally. Ladle into bowls and top each with 1 tablespoon fat-free sour cream, if using.

YIELD: 4 servings

TIP: The salsa I'd recommend is Pace Picante Sauce. Just steer clear of any fancy salsas here, peach or chipotle. You want a plain, tomato-based salsa, not too hot (because it'll get hotter as it cooks and concentrates).

Slow-Cooker Cuban Ropa Vieja

Ropa vieja *means old clothes, presumably because the shredded meat in this Cuban pot roast resembles rags. Don't let the name ruin your appetite. Just think of the old fat clothes you'll be shedding as you drop pounds and pounds of weight on the 17 Day Diet. Ropa vieja is one of my favorite dishes.*

INGREDIENTS

1¼ pound flank steak, trimmed

1 medium red onion, halved through the stem and thinly sliced

1 medium red bell pepper, stemmed, seeded, and thinly sliced

1 medium green bell pepper, stemmed, seeded, and thinly sliced

2 minced medium garlic cloves or 2 teaspoons prepared minced garlic

1 teaspoon dried rosemary

1 teaspoon dried oregano

1 teaspoon ground cumin

½ teaspoon salt

½ teaspoon black pepper

1½ cups fat-free, low-sodium beef broth

2 tablespoons apple-cider vinegar

1 tablespoon reduced-sodium tomato paste

Hot red-pepper sauce, to taste

1 tablespoon packed Cilantro leaves, optional

DIRECTIONS

1. Place the flank steak in the bottom of a 5- to 6-quart slow cooker. Place the onion, bell pepper, garlic, rosemary, oregano, cumin, salt, and pepper over and around the meat. Whisk the broth, vinegar, and tomato paste in a small bowl; pour over the meat and vegetables.

2. Cover and cook on low until the meat is tender enough to be shredded with a fork, 8 to 10 hours. Use two forks to shred the beef into long, thin strips in the pot. If using, stir in some hot red-pepper sauce and cilantro before serving.

(*continued on next page*)

Slow-Cooker Cuban Ropa Vieja (*cont.*)

YIELD: 4 servings

TIPS: To save time, use 2 cups of frozen bell pepper strips in place of the two bell peppers. No need to thaw them. To make this dish on the stovetop, place the beef in a Dutch oven, then add all the ingredients as directed in the recipe. Bring to a simmer over medium-high heat, then reduce the heat to low, cover, and simmer slowly until the meat is tender enough to be shredded with a fork, about 2½ to 3 hours.

Tuscan Pork Tenderloin

I love one-pot meals like this one. Most of my food groups gather in one pan, and that means fewer dishes to wash! The tenderloin is the leanest cut of pork, and is as lean as a skinless chicken breast, and thus a great choice for Cycle 2.

INGREDIENTS

1 tablespoon olive oil

1 pound Brussels sprouts, stems trimmed

4 medium red-skinned potatoes, quartered

1 garlic head, stemmed, broken into cloves, but not peeled

1 tablespoon salt-free Italian spice mix or seasoning blend

1 teaspoon finely grated lemon zest

½ teaspoon salt

1¼-pounds pork tenderloin

1 tablespoon lemon juice

DIRECTIONS

1. Position a rack in the center of the oven and preheat to 375°F.

2. Place the Brussels sprouts, potatoes, and garlic cloves in a large roasting pan or the oven's broiler pan. Toss with the olive oil, then roast for 25 minutes.

3. Meanwhile, mix the spice or seasoning blend, lemon zest, and salt in a small bowl. Pat and smooth this mixture all over the tenderloin.

4. Move the vegetables to the sides of the pan without mounding them; set the tenderloin in the center of the pan. Roast for another 20 minutes.

5. Turn the pork; toss the vegetables. Continue roasting until the meat is cooked through and the potatoes are tender, 15 to 20 additional minutes. Transfer the pork to a carving or cutting board. While the roasting pan is still hot, add the lemon juice and stir

(continued on next page)

Tuscan Pork Tenderloin (*cont.*)

to scrape up any browned bits and coat the vegetables. Carve the pork into ½-inch-thick rounds to serve with the vegetables.

YIELD: 4 servings

TIP: Eat this by squeezing the warm garlic pulp out of the papery hulls and onto the vegetables and pork; it's a sort of roasted-garlic spread. You should probably wait about 10 minutes before serving to let the garlic cool enough to be handled.

Brown Rice Biryani

Biryani *is an Indian, Middle Eastern, and Asian dish made with rice and vegetables. It comes from the Persian word for roasted. You'll fall in love with this dish, especially after you see how little prep time is involved.*

INGREDIENTS

2 pounds frozen mixed vegetables

1 medium garlic clove, minced, or 1 teaspoon prepared minced garlic

1 tablespoon prepared minced ginger

1 cup fat-free, low-sodium chicken broth

½ cup plain, low-fat yogurt

1½ tablespoons curry powder

¼ cup minced cilantro leaves

1 tablespoon lemon juice

2 cups cooked long-grain brown rice, preferably basmati

Vegetable cooking spray

DIRECTIONS

1. Mix the vegetables, garlic, ginger, broth, yogurt, and curry powder in a large saucepan. Set over medium heat and bring to a simmer, stirring occasionally. Cover, reduce the heat to low, and cook for 10 minutes, stirring once in a while.

2. Meanwhile, position a rack in the center of the oven and preheat to 375°F.

3. Stir the cilantro and lemon juice into the vegetable mixture. Pour into a 9-inch square baking pan. Spread the vegetables out evenly, then top with the cooked rice in a solid, fairly compact layer. Spray the top of the rice lightly with nonstick cooking spray; cover the baking dish tightly with aluminum foil.

4. Bake for 20 minutes. Remove the foil and continue baking until the rice dries out and gets a little crispy, about 10 more minutes. Cool for 5 minutes before serving.

(continued on next page)

Brown Rice Biryani (*cont.*)

YIELD: 4 servings

Make Your Own Curry Blend
Mix these spices in a small bowl:
1 tablespoon ground coriander
1 tablespoon turmeric
1 tablespoon ground ginger
1 teaspoon ground fenugreek
1 teaspoon ground mace
1 teaspoon salt
½ teaspoon ground cloves
½ teaspoon ground cinnamon
½ teaspoon ground cumin
Up to ½ teaspoon cayenne
Use in place of bottled curry powder; store in a sealed jar or small plastic container in a cool, dark place for up to 1 year.

TIP: Traditionally, a biryani is served by turning the whole casserole out onto a big platter, the rice now on the bottom, the veggies on top. You can do that here—or just scoop it out servings from the baking pan to plates.

Easy Succotash

Sold in cans since the nineteenth century, succotash is a corn-based dish with other veggies added in, including lima beans. In place of lima beans, we substituted high-protein edamame.

INGREDIENTS

- 1 tablespoon olive oil
- 1 medium yellow onion, chopped
- 2 cups frozen corn kernels
- 1 package (10 ounces) frozen shelled edamame or baby green soy beans
- 1 medium red bell pepper, stemmed, seeded, and cut into thin strips
- 1 medium garlic clove, minced, or 1 teaspoon prepared minced garlic
- 1 tablespoon Southern or Cajun seasoning mix or spice blend
- ½ cup fat-free, low-sodium chicken broth
- 1 tablespoon apple-cider vinegar

DIRECTIONS

1. Swirl the olive oil in a large, preferably nonstick, skillet; set over medium heat for 1 minute. Add the onion; cook until softened, about 3 minutes, stirring occasionally.

2. Add corn, edamame, bell pepper, and garlic; cook, stirring often, until hot, about 4 minutes. Add the seasoning, then pour in the broth. Cook until liquid has almost evaporated, about 7 minutes. Remove the skillet from heat and stir in vinegar.

YIELD: 4 servings

TIPS: To save time, use 1 cup frozen bell pepper strips instead of the whole bell pepper. You can the remainder of the succotash in the fridge and use as a filling for an egg/egg white omelet or warm up and use as a topping for scrambled eggs.

Microwaved Mashed Potatoes

Everyone loves mashed potatoes. The trouble is, you can't eat traditional mashed potatoes on most diets. Those delicious lumps of carbs can turn into unsightly lumps on your hips and thighs. Not so with this recipe! The addition of fat-free sour cream to delectable Yukon Gold potatoes makes these mashed potatoes taste like their fattening counterparts. Enjoy!

INGREDIENTS

4 medium yellow-fleshed potatoes, such as Yukon Golds

¼ cup fat-free, low-sodium chicken broth

2 tablespoons fat-free sour cream

1 tablespoon Dijon mustard

1 tablespoon minced or dried chives, optional

DIRECTIONS

1. Place the potatoes in a medium, microwave-safe bowl. Cover tightly with plastic wrap; make a 1-inch slit in the wrap. Alternatively, use a microwave-safe plastic bowl with a lid; open the small vent hole in the lid.

2. Microwave on high for 8 minutes. Remove the bowl from the microwave, and set aside, covered, for 5 minutes.

3. Uncover and add the broth, sour cream, mustard, and chives, if desired. Mash with a potato masher or a hand mixer until fairly smooth. (Add a little more broth if looser mashed potatoes are desired.)

YIELD: 4 servings

> **TIPS:** The trick here is threefold: the potatoes must not be pricked or poked, the seal on the bowl must be tight, and you can *only* use yellow-fleshed potatoes, like Yukon Golds. Baking or red-skinned potatoes don't have the right moisture/starch ratio to work in the microwave this way.

Pumpkin Polenta

Polenta is the Italian version of cornmeal mush. Cooking polenta used to be time-consuming, requiring constant stirring for almost an hour to make it smooth. Now, with instant polenta, it's a snap, and worth doing. Polenta pairs well with almost everything; here we've added pumpkin, a superfood packed with antioxidants. Pumpkin isn't just for pies anymore!

INGREDIENTS

- 3 cups fat-free, low-sodium chicken broth
- 1¼ cups canned pumpkin puree (do not use canned pumpkin pie filling)
- 1 teaspoon ground cumin
- ½ teaspoon cinnamon
- ½ teaspoon salt
- ½ teaspoon black pepper
- ¼ teaspoon cayenne, optional
- 1 cup instant polenta

DIRECTIONS

1. Put the broth, pumpkin puree, cumin, cinnamon, salt, pepper, and cayenne, if using, in a large saucepan. Set over medium-high heat; whisk occasionally until the pumpkin dissolves and the mixture comes to a simmer.

2. Reduce the heat to medium-low. Whisk in the polenta. Continue stirring until thick and creamy, about 3 minutes.

YIELD: 4 servings

TIPS: A whisk is pretty crucial here to keep the polenta creamy. A wooden spoon will give you lumpier polenta, which is not the worst thing in the world but not the most desirable, either. As a variation, try adding 2 ounces of finely grated fat-free cheese to the polenta, stirring it in at the end, after the pan is off the heat.

Mushroom Barley Sauté

Barley may be one of the oldest grains on earth. It was first used by the Egyptians ten thousand years ago, and brought to America by Christopher Columbus in 1494. Even so, it's not as popular in the United States as oats or rice. As a physician, I'm pushing barley because it can help prevent a lot of health conditions, ranging from balanced blood sugar levels to obesity to cardiovascular disease and cancer. Why is barley so beneficial? It's high in phytochemicals, *which help ward off disease, and it is packed with soluble fiber, know to lower diabetes risk and reduce total blood cholesterol levels. Barley is truly a natural medicine.*

INGREDIENTS

1 cup quick-cooking barley

Nonstick cooking spray

4 medium scallions, thinly sliced

8 ounces white button or cremini mushrooms, sliced thin

1 teaspoon dried thyme

½ teaspoon black pepper

1 tablespoon Worcestershire sauce

DIRECTIONS

1. Bring 2 cups water to a boil in a medium saucepan set over high heat. Stir in the barley. Cover, reduce heat to low, and simmer slowly for 10 minutes. Remove from the heat and let stand, covered, until the water is fully absorbed, about 5 minutes.

2. Spray a large skillet with nonstick cooking spray; set over medium heat for 1 minute. Add the scallions and mushrooms; cook, stirring often, until the mushrooms are tender, 8 to 10 minutes.

3. Stir in the thyme and pepper; cook for 20 seconds. Add the cooked barley and the Worcestershire sauce; cook, stirring constantly, until heated through, about 1 minute.

YIELD: 4 servings

TIP: The barley can be cooked in advance. Keep it in the fridge in a covered container for up to 3 days. Warm in a microwave for 1 minute on high before adding it to the skillet.

Also, this can be used as a bed for the falafel patties in the Falafel Salad (page 71).

White Bean and Red Pepper Dip

You've got the munchies and just have to have some salt and crunch. Hold it—I don't want you to munch on chips and dip! Be willing to push that junk aside. It's what you choose for a snack that makes a difference in your weight loss. Snacking on healthy foods can be a good and convenient way to satisfy your cravings, while giving your body a nutritional boost. Try this dip the next time you have a snack attack.

INGREDIENTS
1 can (15 ounces) white beans, drained and rinsed
1 roasted red pepper, cut into 3 pieces
¼ cup yogurt cheese
1 garlic clove, peeled
1 tablespoon lemon juice
½ teaspoon salt
½ teaspoon ground black pepper

DIRECTIONS
Place all the ingredients in a food processor fitted with the chopping blade; process until creamy, scraping down the inside of the bowl once or twice.

YIELD: 4 servings

TIPS: Serve with cut-up celery, cucumber rounds, baby carrots, and broccoli florets. Bring those to work or school in a separate container for a quick lunch.

Dip stores well in a sealed container in the fridge for up to 3 days.

Spiced Edamame

It's no secret that to drop pounds or tackle our cholesterol, we have to watch fat and carbs, eat more veggies, and turn cheesecake into a treat, not an everyday treat. But have you ever wondered, while you're getting trim and healthy, how to eat to slow aging and stay young? A great anti-aging food is the bean, including edamame (soy beans). This miracle veggie is loaded with heart-healthy folic acid and fiber to keep you slim. Plus, it's digested slowly and enters the bloodstream gradually, which minimizes the spikes in blood sugar that can lead to cravings and weight gain. A few weeks from now, when you're slimmer and sexier, you'll be glad you put this version of edamame on your plate.

INGREDIENTS

1 (1 pound) bag frozen edamame or baby green soy beans in their pods

1 teaspoon salt

½ teaspoon ground coriander

½ teaspoon dried ginger

½ teaspoon red-pepper flakes, optional

DIRECTIONS

1. Bring a large pot of water to a boil over high heat. Add the edamame. Boil for 8 minutes. Drain in a colander. Lay some paper towels on your work surface; pour the edamame onto them. Pat dry.

2. Place the cooked edamame in a bowl; add the salt, coriander, ginger, and red-pepper flakes, if using. Toss well.

YIELD: 4 servings

TIPS: As you know, you don't eat the pods. You scrape the beans out through their pods with your teeth, getting some of the spice mixture as you do. You can also use 2½ teaspoons of the curry blend we made for the Brown Rice Biryani (page 87).

Mexican Chocolate Pudding

Chocolate is heavenly. Chocolate rules. Chocolate, my friends, is a terrible thing to shun on a diet. With this recipe, you can have your chocolate and eat it, too. It's a pudding made with high-protein, super-nutritious tofu. And if you think you don't like tofu, get over it. Tofu takes on whatever flavor it is paired with, including chocolate!

INGREDIENTS
   12.3 ounce package silken extra-firm tofu
   5 tablespoons unsweetened cocoa powder
   3 tablespoons sugar-free chocolate-flavored syrup
   2 teaspoons Truvia
   ½ teaspoon almond extract
   ½ teaspoon cinnamon
   ¼ teaspoon or less cayenne, optional

DIRECTIONS
Place all the ingredients in a large food processor. Cover and process until smooth, about 1 minute, scraping down the inside of the bowl at least once. Divide into four ramekins or small bowls; serve immediately or refrigerate.

YIELD: 4 servings

TIP: It's important to get the silken extra-firm tofu. Mori-Nu sells it in packages that are shelf-stable, no refrigeration needed. Please use cocoa powder, not hot cocoa mix. The pudding is not pourable but very thick. You will have to scrape it out of the food processor. A blender will not work because the tofu is so thick.

Grilled Spiced Peaches

Did someone say peaches? Grab some fresh ones and start cooking. Bonus points if the juice drips down your hand like water over Niagara Falls when you slice them. Peaches are rich in potassium and vitamins A, B, and C, too. At the grocery store or farmer's markets, look for peaches that give with soft pressure, have a nice aroma, and no dark or mushy spots. If they aren't fully ripe, place the peaches in a brown paper bag at room temperature for a day or two to soften.

INGREDIENTS

4 teaspoons flaxseed oil

4 large ripe peaches, halved and pitted

1½ teaspoons apple-pie spice blend

1 teaspoon Truvia

½ cup sugar-free, low-fat raspberry yogurt

DIRECTIONS

1. Heat a large grill pan over medium-high heat. Alternatively, prepare and heat an outdoor grill for direct, high-heat cooking.

2. Brush ½ teaspoon oil on the cut side of each peach. Mix the spice blend and Truvia in a small bowl; sprinkle evenly over the cut side of the peach halves.

3. Set the peaches cut side down on the grill pan or on the grill's cooking grate directly over the heat. Grill until golden brown, about 2 minutes. Turn with a wide, flat spatula or tongs; continue grilling for 1 minute. Transfer to plates, cut side up. Put 1 tablespoon yogurt in the center of each peach half.

YIELD: 4 servings

TIP: Best to get freestone peaches, not cling, so that you can remove pits easily.

17 Sample Cycle 2 Menus

Here are examples of how you can create your daily menu using the preceding recipes during the Activate Cycle.

Day 1

Breakfast

☐ 1 *Dr. Mike's Power Cookie*

☐ 1 fresh peach, sliced

☐ 1 cup green tea

Lunch

☐ 1 serving *Smoked Turkey and Lentil Salad*

☐ 6 ounces sugar-free, fruit-flavored yogurt

Dinner

☐ 1 serving *Curried Poached Halibut*

☐ Steamed veggies

Snack

☐ 1 serving *Super Strawberry Smoothie*

Day 2

Breakfast

☐ 1 serving *Snappy Eggs*

☐ ½ grapefruit, or other fresh fruit

☐ 1 cup green tea

Lunch

☐ 1 serving *California Tuna Salad*

☐ 1 cup green tea

Dinner

☐ 1 serving *Tandoori Chicken Breasts*

☐ 1 cup green tea

Snacks

☐ 6 ounces nonfat yogurt, sweetened with Truvia or a tablespoon of sugar-free fruit jam or other probiotic serving

☐ 1 serving of fruit from the Cycle 1 list

Day 3

Breakfast

☐ 1 serving *Eggs, Lox, and Onions*

☐ ½ grapefruit, or other fresh fruit

☐ 1 cup green tea

Lunch

☐ 1 serving *Easy Chicken Posole*

☐ 6 ounces sugar-free, fruit-flavored yogurt

☐ 1 cup green tea

Dinner

☐ 1 serving *Slow-Cooker Cuban Ropa Vieja*

☐ 1 cup green tea

Snacks

☐ 1 cup fresh raspberries or other in-season fruit with 6 ounces sugar-free, fruit-flavored yogurt

☐ 1 serving *White Bean and Red Pepper Dip*

Day 4

Breakfast

☐ 1 serving *Mushroom Spinach Frittata*

☐ ½ grapefruit or other fresh fruit in season

☐ 1 cup green tea

Lunch

☐ 1 large bowl of *Chicken-Vegetable Soup*

☐ 1 cup green tea

Dinner

☐ Plenty of roasted turkey breast or turkey tenderloin, steamed carrots, and steamed asparagus.

☐ 1 cup green tea

Snacks

☐ 6 ounces nonfat yogurt, sweetened with Truvia or a tablespoon of sugar-free fruit jam

☐ *Kefir Smoothie*

Day 5

Breakfast

- ☐ 1 serving *Weekend Morning Grits Casserole*
- ☐ 1 fresh peach, sliced
- ☐ 1 cup green tea

Lunch

- ☐ 1 serving *Crab Tabouleh*
- ☐ 1 cup green tea

Dinner

- ☐ 1 serving *Stewed Mussels*
- ☐ 1 cup green tea

Snacks

- ☐ 1 cup blueberries with 6 ounces sugar-free fruit-flavored yogurt
- ☐ 6 ounces sugar-free, fruit-flavored yogurt or 1 cup kefir

Day 6

Breakfast

- ☐ 6 ounces plain low-fat yogurt, mixed with 1 cup berries, or other fruit on the Cycle 1 list sweetened with Truvia or a tablespoon of sugar-free fruit jam.
- ☐ 1 cup green tea

Lunch

- ☐ Grilled chicken breast with tossed salad drizzled with 1 tablespoon of olive or flaxseed oil and 2 tablespoons balsamic vinegar
- ☐ 1 cup green tea

Dinner

- ☐ 1 serving *Curried Poached Halibut*
- ☐ 1 cup green tea

Snacks

- ☐ 1 serving *Grilled Spiced Peaches*
- ☐ Probiotic serving

Day 7

Breakfast

☐ 1 serving *Snappy Eggs*

☐ 1 orange or other fresh fruit in season

☐ 1 cup green tea

Lunch

☐ 1 serving *Fast and Easy Chili*

☐ Large tossed salad with 1 tablespoon olive oil mixed with 2 tablespoons vinegar and seasoning

☐ 1 cup green tea

Dinner

☐ 1 serving *Turkey and Bulgur Meatloaf*

☐ 1 serving *Spicy Green Beans*

☐ 1 cup green tea

Snacks

☐ *Kefir Smoothie*

☐ 6 ounces sugar-free, fruit-flavored yogurt

Day 8

Breakfast

- ☐ 6 ounces plain low-fat yogurt, mixed with 1 cup berries, or other fruit on the Cycle 1 list, sweetened with 1 packet of Truvia or a tablespoon of sugar-free fruit jam.
- ☐ 1 cup green tea

Lunch

- ☐ 1 serving *Lemon-Pepper Salmon Salad in Tomato Cups*
- ☐ 1 cup green tea

Dinner

- ☐ Turkey burgers made with lean ground turkey
- ☐ Steamed vegetables (choose from Cycle 1 vegetables)
- ☐ Side salad drizzled with drizzled with 1 tablespoon olive or flax-seed oil, mixed with 2 tablespoons balsamic vinegar and seasonings
- ☐ 1 cup green tea

Snack

- ☐ 1 serving *Berry Frozen Yogurt*

Day 9

Breakfast

- □ ½ cup Breakstone LiveActive cottage cheese
- □ 1 medium pear, sliced
- □ 1 cup green tea

Lunch

- □ Grilled chicken breast
- □ 1 serving *Pumpkin Polenta*
- □ 1 cup green tea

Dinner

- □ Grilled salmon
- □ Steamed broccoli
- □ 1 serving *Mexican Chocolate Pudding*
- □ 1 cup green tea

Snacks

- □ 1 medium apple
- □ 6 ounces sugar-free, fruit-flavored yogurt

Day 10

Breakfast

☐ 1 serving *Spanish Omelet*

☐ ½ grapefruit or 1 medium orange

☐ 1 cup green tea

Lunch

☐ 1 serving *Creamy Smoked Salmon Rolls*

☐ 1 cup green tea

Dinner

☐ Plenty of roasted turkey breast or turkey tenderloin, steamed carrots, and steamed asparagus

☐ 1 cup green tea

Snacks

☐ 1 piece fresh fruit

☐ 6 ounces nonfat yogurt

Day 11

Breakfast

☐ 1 serving *Kefir Smoothie*

☐ 1 cup green tea

Lunch

☐ Plenty of broiled hamburger

☐ 1 serving *Microwaved Mashed Potatoes*

Dinner

☐ 1 serving *Tuscan Pork Tenderloin*

☐ Steamed asparagus

☐ Large tossed salad with 1 tablespoon olive oil mixed with 2 tablespoons vinegar and seasoning

Snacks

☐ 1 medium orange

☐ 6 ounces sugar-free, fruit-flavored yogurt

Day 12

Breakfast

☐ 1 serving *Yogurt Fruitshake*

☐ 1 cup green tea

Lunch

☐ 1 serving *Super Salad*

☐ 1 cup green tea

Dinner

☐ Steamed flounder or sole with lemon pepper

☐ Steamed broccoli

☐ 1 cup green tea

Snacks

☐ 1 medium apple, or other fruit in season

☐ 1 serving *Berry Frozen Yogurt*

Day 13

Breakfast

☐ 1 *Dr. Mike's Power Cookie*

☐ 1 medium peach, sliced

☐ 1 cup green tea

Lunch

☐ Fruit salad: ½ cup LiveActive Breakstone cottage cheese with ½ cup diced strawberries and ½ cup diced peach served on a generous bed of lettuce

☐ 1 cup green tea

Dinner

☐ 1 serving *Roasted Shrimp and Broccoli*

☐ 1 cup green tea

Snacks

☐ 1 serving *Yogurt Fruitshake*

☐ 1 serving *Berry Frozen Yogurt*

Day 14

Breakfast

☐ 1 serving *Peach Melba Smoothie*

☐ 1 cup green tea

Lunch

☐ 1 serving *Super Salad*

☐ 1 cup green tea

Dinner

☐ 1 serving *Blackened Catfish* with liberal amounts of any Cycle 1 vegetables, steamed or raw

☐ 1 cup green tea

Snacks

☐ 6 ounces sugar-free fruit-flavored yogurt, or 1 cup plain low-fat yogurt, sweetened with Truvia or a tablespoon of sugar-free fruit jam

☐ 1 serving of fruit

Day 15

Breakfast

- ☐ ½ cup cooked oatmeal
- ☐ 6 ounces sugar-free, fruit-flavored yogurt
- ☐ 1 cup green tea

Lunch

- ☐ 1 serving *Cantonese Stir-Fried Shrimp*
- ☐ 1 cup green tea

Dinner

- ☐ 1 serving *Turkey and Bulgur Meatloaf*
- ☐ 1 cup green tea

Snacks

- ☐ 1 medium apple or pear
- ☐ 2nd probiotic serving

Day 16

Breakfast

- ☐ 2 scrambled egg whites
- ☐ ½ grapefruit or other fresh fruit in season
- ☐ 1 cup green tea

Lunch

- ☐ 1 large bowl of *Chicken-Vegetable Soup*
- ☐ 1 cup green tea

Dinner

- ☐ 1 serving *Stir-Fried Chicken and Cucumbers*
- ☐ 1 cup green tea

Snacks

- ☐ 1 cup of fresh berries
- ☐ 6 ounces nonfat yogurt, sweetened with Truvia or a tablespoon of sugar-free fruit jam

NOTES

Day 17

Breakfast

☐ 1 serving *Eggs, Lox, and Onions*

☐ 1 cup fresh berries

☐ 1 cup green tea

Lunch

☐ 1 serving *Italian Shrimp and White Bean Salad*

☐ 1 cup green tea

Dinner

☐ 1 serving *Bavarian Chicken Breasts*

☐ 1 cup green tea

Snacks

☐ 1 medium orange or nectarine

☐ 2nd probiotic serving

RECIPES

Cycle 3—Achieve

GOAL: To develop good eating habits through the reintroduction of additional foods and move you closer to your goal weight.

Better Migas

I love migas (MEE-gahs), a spicy concoction of tortillas scrambled with eggs, peppers, and beans, topped with salsa. On a good morning, I prefer my migas with a shot of hot sauce. This recipe has all the robust flavor of traditional migas without the fat and calories. It's high in fiber, too, thanks to the addition of pinto beans. Eggs, of course, are the ultimate protein: They digest easily, help prevent fat deposits, and are good for memory and concentration.

INGREDIENTS

1 can (15 ounces) pinto beans, drained and rinsed

1 canned chipotle chili in adobo sauce, stemmed

2 tablespoons lime juice

1 tablespoon chili powder

½ teaspoon garlic powder

½ teaspoon salt

Two 10-inch whole-wheat tortillas

Nonstick cooking spray

2 large eggs

¼ cup prepared salsa

2 tablespoons low-fat Cheddar cheese

DIRECTIONS

1. Place the pinto beans, chipotle, lime juice, 2 tablespoons water, chili powder, garlic powder, and salt in a large processor. Cover and process until fairly smooth, like refried beans, scraping down the inside of the bowl once or twice. Set aside.

2. Set a large nonstick skillet over medium heat for 1 minute. Add the tortillas one at a time; cook, turning once, until warmed and a little browned, about 1 minute. Transfer to two plates. Spread each of the tortillas with ¼ cup of the bean mixture. Wipe out the skillet.

(continued on next page)

Better Migas (*cont.*)

3. Spray the nonstick skillet with nonstick cooking spray; set over the heat for 1 minute. Crack the eggs into the skillet. Cook until the whites are set but the yolks are soft, about 3 minutes, flipping after 2 minutes. (For sunny-side up eggs, cook for about 2½ minutes without flipping; for harder cooked yolks, cook 1 minute longer after flipping.) Use a large spatula to set a fried egg on each tortilla. Top each with 2 tablespoons salsa and 1 tablespoon shredded cheese.

YIELD: 2 servings

> **TIPS:** Using this recipe, you've essentially made mock refried beans, much lower in fat but just as tasty. It'll make more than you need, which is a good thing, because the leftovers can be served as a dip or as a side dish. Store it, covered, in the fridge. It can be heated in the microwave for a minute or two. Make sure you use 1 canned chipotle in adobo sauce, not 1 can of chipotles in adobo sauce. Canned chipotles in adobo sauce are found in most supermarkets near the canned refried beans and other Mexican foods.

Slow-Cooker Brown Rice Congee

Doctors don't have a lot of time to read, but when we do read, we read medical journals, which sounds kind of boring. The last journal I read was the Journal of Chinese Medicine, *in which I learned about* congee, *a creamy rice soup that is a traditional breakfast food in China. It sounded perfect for the 17 Day Diet, so I include my brown-rice version here. The article, by the way, linked eating congee to living longer. I suppose that means you can enjoy your fit, trim body longer by adding this tasty, light, and healthy breakfast food to your menu.*

INGREDIENTS

8 cups vegetable broth

1 cup medium-grain brown rice, such as brown Arborio rice

1 tablespoon minced peeled fresh ginger or 1 tablespoon prepared minced ginger

Suggested garnishes

Thinly sliced scallions

Chopped, skinless, boneless chicken breast

Chopped, cooked shrimp

Diced firm tofu

Dry roasted salted peanuts

Asian hot sauce, such as sambal olek or sriracha

DIRECTIONS

1. Stir the broth, rice, and ginger in a 5- to 6-quart slow cooker. Cover and cook on low until creamy and porridgelike, about 10 hours.

2. To serve, ladle 1-cup servings into bowls. Sprinkle with small amounts of one or more garnishes. Or skip the toppings altogether and enjoy the congee as a hot, savory, breakfast cereal on its own.

YIELD: 8 servings

(continued on next page)

Slow-Cooker Brown Rice Congee (*cont.*)

> **TIPS:** Leftovers can be refrigerated then reheated in a microwave or a small pot the next day. If too stiff after refrigerating, loosen the dish with a little extra broth or water before reheating. This is a great recipe for weekend company or a holiday breakfast alternative.

Breakfast Pizza Bagels

Left-over pizza for breakfast? Admit it: You've eaten it. Maybe not the best choice but it does hit the spot occasionally, especially when there's nothing else in the fridge. Not to worry. This nutritious, filling recipe now makes it legitimate to eat pizza for breakfast.

INGREDIENTS

1 whole-grain bagel, split in half

4 ounces reduced-fat Swiss cheese, thinly sliced

2 teaspoons minced chives or the green part of a scallion

4 thin tomato slices

½ teaspoon salt

DIRECTIONS

1. Position an oven rack 4 to 6 inches from the broiler; preheat the broiler. Set the bagel halves cut side up on a baking sheet. Broil until brown and toasty, about 2 minutes.

2. Remove the baking sheet from the oven; leave the broiler on. Top each bagel half with 2 ounces sliced cheese, 1 teaspoon minced chives, 2 tomato slices, and ¼ teaspoon salt. Broil until the tomatoes are bubbling and the cheese has melted, about 2 minutes.

YIELD: 2 servings

TIPS: You don't want seeds or other toppings on the bagel because they can burn in the intense broiler heat. Use a large globe or slicing tomato for the best slices. Don't like chives? Try some stemmed thyme leaves or minced oregano leaves.

Banana Chocolate Smoothie

If you're craving something chocolaty, why not set your sights on something truly worth coveting? I'm talking about a delicious, creamy chocolate smoothie to kick-start your day. With the addition of a banana and silken tofu, this is one smoothie that tastes decadent, but has huge health payoffs: lots of fiber, low in fat, and if you opt for soy milk, it's dairy-, gluten-, and lactose-free.

INGREDIENTS

1 small banana, peeled and cut into 1-inch pieces
½ cup soft silken tofu
½ cup soy milk or low-fat milk
3 tablespoons sugar-free chocolate-flavored syrup
1 teaspoon Truvia

DIRECTIONS

Place all the ingredients in a blender. Cover and blend until smooth, turning off the machine and scraping down the inside of the container at least once.

YIELD: 1 serving (can be doubled)

> **TIPS:** Want it colder? Add an ice cube. Want more texture? Add 1 tablespoon toasted wheat germ.

White Bean and Oat Burgers

There are plenty of meat substitutes like vegetarian and vegan burgers in the marketplace, and for the most part, they taste pretty good. Or least I thought so, until I tasted these. Delicious. You won't be asking "Where's the beef?" you'll be asking, "Who needs the beef?"

INGREDIENTS

1 can (15 ounces) white beans, drained and rinsed

½ cup regular rolled oats (do not use quick-cooking or steel-cut oats)

2 ounces (about 24) whole roasted almonds (do not use salted almonds)

1 large egg

1 tablespoon minced sage leaves or 1½ teaspoons dried sage

1 teaspoon salt

½ teaspoon ground black pepper

¼ teaspoon garlic powder

¼ teaspoon onion powder

1 tablespoon olive oil

4 whole-wheat pita pockets

Chopped iceberg lettuce

½ cup bottled low-fat ranch dressing

DIRECTIONS

1. Place the beans, oats, almonds, egg, sage, salt, pepper, garlic powder, and onion powder in a food processor fitted with the chopping blade. Cover and process until pasty, scraping down the inside of the bowl once or twice.

2. Scrape down and remove the chopping blade. Use wet hands to scoop up and pat the mixture into four equal patties, each about 5 inches in diameter.

3. Heat the oil in a large nonstick skillet over medium heat. Slip the patties into the skillet and cook until browned and firm, about 8 minutes, turning once. Serve the patties in the pita pockets, each

(continued on next page)

White Bean and Oat Burgers (*cont.*)

stuffed with chopped lettuce and drizzled with 2 tablespoons ranch dressing.

YIELD: 4 servings

> **TIPS:** The patties can be cooked and saved, covered, in the fridge. To recrisp them, heat in a dry skillet over medium heat, about 4 minutes, turning once, or place them on a baking sheet and bake for about 10 minutes in a 350°F oven.

Open-Faced Reuben

Every so often I get a real craving for a Reuben sandwich. However, the traditional sandwich includes high-fat Russian or Thousand Island dressing, corned beef, and Swiss cheese, and is fried in butter. We slimmed down the Reuben by using low-fat turkey pastrami, low-fat Russian dressing, and low-fat Swiss cheese. Instead of frying the sandwich in butter, you carefully broil it. And, let me tell you, this retooled Reuben is magnificent.

INGREDIENTS

2 slices pumpernickel bread

2 tablespoons low-fat prepared Russian dressing

2 ounces low-fat turkey pastrami, thinly sliced

4 thin tomato slices

⅔ cup drained and rinsed sauerkraut

3 ounces low-fat Swiss cheese, sliced thin

DIRECTIONS

1. Position the oven rack 4 to 6 inches from the broiler. Lay the bread slices on a baking sheet; toast until crunchy, about 3 minutes, turning once. Remove from the oven; leave the broiler on.

2. Spread each slice with 1 tablespoon Russian dressing. Top with 1 ounce turkey pastrami, 2 tomato slices, ⅓ cup sauerkraut, and 1½ ounces cheese. Broil until the cheese has melted and is beginning to brown, about 3 minutes.

YIELD: 2 servings (can be doubled)

TIPS: The best sauerkraut is found in bags or jars in the refrigerator section or deli case of your supermarket. Drain the sauerkraut well, even squeezing it a bit by handfuls over the sink. You don't want excess moisture to make the bread soggy.

Brie and Mango Quesadilla

Gourmet meets Tex-Mex, and it's a marriage made in culinary heaven. And so quick to make. In less than 10 minutes, you've got a meal. Now, that's my kind of lunch.

INGREDIENTS

Two 10-inch whole-wheat tortillas
4 ounces Brie, rind removed
1 large mango, peeled, pitted, and thinly sliced
1 roasted red pepper, cut in half
Nonstick cooking spray

DIRECTIONS

1. Lay one tortilla on a work surface. Spread half the cheese over half the tortilla. Lay half the mango and ½ roasted red pepper over the cheese. Fold the tortilla to make a semicircle. Repeat with the other tortilla.

2. Spray a large nonstick skillet with vegetable cooking spray. Set over medium heat for 1 minute. Add the quesadillas; cook until the tortilla is lightly browned and the cheese has melted, about 4 minutes, turning once.

YIELD: 2 servings (can be doubled)

> **TIPS:** You can find sliced mango in the refrigerator case of the produce section of most supermarkets. One traditional way to make quesadillas is to weigh them down in the skillet, making them flatter and crisper. Weigh them down with a heavy pot lid or even a large saucepan, pressing a bit as it first sits on top of them. Or put a lightweight lid on them and top with a 15-ounce can of beans.

Crab Gazpacho

Gazpacho is the king of cold soups. It brings together a veritable garden of healthy veggies all in one bowl. Ours is souped up with crabmeat for an extra punch of protein, resulting in a complete meal that's healthy, simple, and easy to make.

INGREDIENTS

2 large tomatoes, finely chopped, all juice reserved

1 medium green bell pepper, stemmed, seeded, and finely chopped

1 large carrot, peeled and coarsely shredded

2 celery stalks, finely chopped

½ large cucumber, peeled, seeded, and finely chopped

¼ cup minced red onion

2 tablespoons Worcestershire sauce

1 tablespoon lemon juice

Several dashes hot red-pepper sauce

1 cup pasteurized lump crabmeat

DIRECTIONS

Stir the tomatoes, bell pepper, carrot, celery, cucumber, red onion, Worcestershire sauce, lemon juice, and hot-red-pepper sauce in a medium bowl. Divide between 2 serving bowls; top each with half the crabmeat.

YIELD: 2 servings (can be doubled)

> **TIPS:** The trick here is to finely chop the vegetables so they're all about the same size, so that you can have different flavors and textures in every spoonful.
>
> The soup keeps well in the fridge, covered, for up to 3 days. Can be served cold. If taking for lunch, carry the crabmeat in a separate container, then add when you are ready to eat.

Spinach Mushroom Salad with Warm Bacon Dressing

Most versions of this popular salad are rather weighty due to the amount of bacon used. This recipe relies on a lower-fat alternative: turkey bacon. The addition of feta cheese and mushrooms adds to this salad's tastiness.

INGREDIENTS

4 cups baby spinach leaves

4 ounces thinly sliced white button or cremini mushrooms

2 teaspoons olive oil

4 slices turkey bacon, chopped

1 tablespoon minced shallot

1 tablespoon apple-cider vinegar

1 teaspoon Dijon mustard

2 ounces feta

½ teaspoon ground black pepper

DIRECTIONS

1. Toss the spinach and mushrooms in a large bowl. Set aside.

2. Heat the oil in a nonstick skillet over medium heat. Add the bacon; cook, stirring often, until crisp, about 3 minutes. Add the shallots; stir over the heat for 30 seconds to soften them. Stir in the vinegar and mustard. Pour the warm dressing over the spinach and mushrooms; toss well.

3. Divide the salad between 2 plates. Top each with half the feta and the black pepper.

YIELD: 2 servings (can be doubled)

TIP: The hot dressing should wilt the spinach leaves a bit.

Tex-Mex Millet Salad

Here's one of the healthiest and highest fiber salads you'll ever make. It spotlights two unusual ingredients: Nutty-tasting millet, a nutritious gluten-free grain that's a cereal a staple in Africa, Asia, and India; and jicama (pronounced hee-ka-ma), a low-calorie root vegetable with an applelike texture. Jicama contains a group of fibers known as fructans, *specifically* inulin, *which helps promote bone and digestive health. Added to the salad are other high-fiber goodies: pinto beans, corn, almonds, and plums.*

INGREDIENTS

½ cup millet (do not use millet grits)

1 cup canned pinto beans, drained and rinsed

1 can (4 ounces) chopped roasted green chilies, hot or mild

1 small jicama, peeled and chopped

1 large ripe, red plum, pitted and chopped

½ cup frozen corn kernels, thawed

¼ cup sliced almonds

2 tablespoons lime juice

2 teaspoons chili powder

1 teaspoon olive oil or walnut oil, if desired

DIRECTIONS

1. Bring 1¼ cups water to a boil over high heat. Stir in the millet. Cover, reduce the heat to low, and simmer until the water has been absorbed and the millet is tender, about 25 minutes.

2. Scrape the millet into a large bowl. Stir in the beans, chilies, jicama, plum, corn, almonds, lime juice, chili powder, and oil, if desired.

YIELD: 2 servings (can be doubled)

> **TIP:** Once the millet is cooked, don't let it sit around or it'll start to firm up. Dump it into the bowl and stir in the remaining ingredients to keep the grains separate and soft. Store in a sealed container in the fridge for up to 3 days.

Shrimp Soba Noodle Salad

Pasta salad has a lot of loyal fans, and this recipe will create many more. It's made with soba, a Japanese noodle usually made from buckwheat and wheat flour. Soba noodles are a health food: Thanks to the buckwheat, they contain rutin, *a natural plant compound believed to help reduce blood pressure and strengthen blood vessels. Rutin may even have anticancer properties. The addition of shrimp to this flavorful pasta salad adds low-fat protein to the mix. So use your noodle, your soba noodles, that is, and enjoy an Asian rendition of a pasta salad.*

INGREDIENTS

2 tablespoons unseasoned rice vinegar

1 tablespoon light soy sauce

2 teaspoons toasted sesame oil

1 teaspoon peeled, minced fresh ginger

1 cup cooked soba noodles

6 ounces cooked shrimp, chopped

1 large carrot, coarsely shredded

1 small red bell pepper, stemmed, seeded, and thinly sliced

2 medium scallions, thinly sliced

2 tablespoons minced cilantro leaves

DIRECTIONS

1. Whisk the vinegar, soy sauce, sesame oil, and ginger in a large bowl.

2. Add the noodles, shrimp, carrot, bell pepper, scallions, and cilantro. Toss well.

YIELD: 2 servings (can be doubled)

TIPS: Cook 4 ounces fresh soba noodles in a big pot of boiling water to get 1 cup cooked soba noodles.

Use toasted sesame oil for the most flavor; once opened, store it in the fridge to preserve its freshness. It may solidify somewhat but will regain its liquidity after sitting at room temperature for 10 minutes.

If you're taking this to work, pack the dressing separately, so the vegetables stay fresh and crisp.

Easy Cioppino

There's nothing better than a steaming cup of authentic cioppino (pronounced cha-pe-no), a wonderful fish stew with a rich, spicy tomato base loaded with herbs. I love it. I could bathe in it, and would happily agree to an IV of it, if that's what the doctor ordered, and I'm the doctor. This recipe, usually served in waterside restaurants, is so authentic that I can hear the seagulls in the San Diego Bay. Soup's on!

INGREDIENTS

1 can (28 ounces) diced tomatoes

1 cup vegetable broth

1 medium yellow onion, chopped

1 medium fennel bulb, trimmed and chopped

1 medium green bell pepper, stemmed, seeded, and chopped

2 celery stalks, chopped

1 medium garlic clove, minced, or 1 teaspoon prepared minced garlic

2 teaspoons dried basil

2 teaspoons dried oregano

½ teaspoon red-pepper flakes

½ pound halibut, cut into 1-inch cubes

1 pound mussels, cleaned and debearded

DIRECTIONS

1. Bring the tomatoes, broth, onion, fennel, bell pepper, celery, garlic, basil, oregano, and red-pepper flakes to a simmer in a large saucepan set over high heat. Cover, reduce the heat to very low, and simmer for 30 minutes.

2. Add the halibut and mussels. Cover and continue simmering until the mussels open, about 10 minutes. Discard any mussels that do not open.

YIELD: 4 servings

TIPS: To save time, use 1 cup frozen chopped onion and 1 cup frozen bell pepper strips instead of the fresh vegetables. Thaw the frozen vegetables before using. For information on the cleaning and debearding of mussels, see page 77.

Roasted Trout Almandine

I've eaten a lot of trout Almandine at restaurants, and this version rivals anything I've tasted. It's so moist and flavorful; you'd think the fish had been swimming in a river of butter. No butter is used here, however, so we keep the fat and calories well below stratospheric range.

INGREDIENTS
Nonstick cooking spray
2 small whole trout, boned and cleaned
1 medium lemon, cut into 6 paper-thin slices and 2 wedges
4 fresh thyme sprigs
6 tablespoons sliced almonds
½ teaspoon salt
½ teaspoon black pepper

DIRECTIONS
1. Position a rack in the center of the oven and preheat to 400°F.

2. Spray a roasting pan or the broiler pan with vegetable cooking spray. Lay the trout in the pan; layer the lemon slices and thyme in the body cavity of each of the trout. Place 1 tablespoon sliced almonds in each trout as well. Close the fish and sprinkle the remaining sliced almonds over the top. Season with salt and pepper.

3. Bake until the flesh flakes when pulled with a fork, 12 to 15 minutes. Remove from the oven and squeeze the lemon wedges over the trout and almonds. Cut each trout in half across to serve.

YIELD: 4 servings

> **TIPS:** Make sure you get boned, cleaned trout. Even so, if you're sharing a trout with a child, check for bones, particularly along the dorsal fin along the spine at the top. If you're squeamish, ask the fishmonger to remove the heads for you.

Snapper Veracruz

Red snapper is a white firm-fleshed fish that benefits from a spicy treatment, which this wonderfully rendered dish has. Red Snapper Veracruz style is a classic Mexican dish in which the fish is baked in a zippy sauce made with tomatoes, peppers, and capers. Enjoy!

INGREDIENTS

1 can (28 ounces) diced tomatoes

1 medium red bell pepper, stemmed, cored, and chopped

1 medium green bell pepper, stemmed, cored, and chopped

10 jarred, pickled jalapeño slices, drained and chopped, or to taste

¼ cup chopped fresh parsley leaves

1 tablespoon fresh thyme leaves or 2 teaspoons dried thyme

1 teaspoon drained and rinsed capers, chopped

½ teaspoon salt

Four 4-ounce skinless snapper fillets

DIRECTIONS

1. Bring the tomatoes, bell pepper, jalapeño, parsley, thyme, capers and salt to a simmer in a Dutch oven set over medium-high heat. Cover, reduce the heat to low, and simmer slowly for 20 minutes.

2. Slip the fish fillets into the tomato mixture. Cover and cook until the fish flakes when pierced with a fork, about 10 minutes. Ladle the soup and fish into bowls to serve.

YIELD: 4 servings

TIP: To save time, use 2 cups frozen bell pepper strips, thawed, instead of the two bell peppers. You'll have strips, not chopped bell pepper, but that won't matter much, except the look of the dish.

Broiled Miso-Glazed Salmon

Using a glaze on this favorite fish is a fast way to add flavor without having to marinate the salmon. This sweet-and-sour glaze gets its flavor from soy sauce, no-sugar-added apricot preserves or all-fruit spread, and miso paste. Miso is a mixture of cooked soybeans, salt, a steamed grain, such as rice, wheat, or barley that has been injected with a mold culture to stimulate fermentation. Miso's flavor has been describe in hundreds of ways, including rich, earthy, tangy, beany, nutty, buttery, mushroomy, meaty, and salty.

INGREDIENTS

¼ cup white miso paste

3 tablespoons unseasoned rice vinegar

3 tablespoons light soy sauce

2 tablespoons sugar-free apricot preserves or all-fruit spread

1 tablespoon minced peeled fresh ginger or jarred minced ginger

Four 4-ounce skinless salmon fillets

DIRECTIONS

1. Stir the miso paste, rice vinegar, soy sauce, apricot preserves, and ginger in a large bowl.

2. Spread the miso mixture on both sides of each fillet; place on a baking sheet

3. Position the rack 4 to 6 inches from the broiler; preheat the broiler.

4. Set the tray on the rack and broil for 4 minutes. Use a large spatula to turn the fillets and continue broiling until the salmon flakes when tested with a fork, about 4 more minutes.

YIELD: 4 servings

TIP: There are several kinds of miso; make sure you use the milder white.

Shrimp Vindaloo

Vindaloo is a spicy curry. Grapes counterbalance all the spices, with a flavor combo that will enliven your palate.

INGREDIENTS

1 teaspoon salt

½ teaspoon dry mustard

½ teaspoon ground coriander

½ teaspoon ground cumin

½ teaspoon ground ginger

½ teaspoon turmeric

¼ to ½ teaspoon cayenne

¼ teaspoon ground cinnamon

⅛ teaspoon ground cloves

1½ tablespoons red-wine vinegar

Nonstick cooking spray

1 large yellow onion, chopped

3 tablespoons peeled minced fresh ginger or prepared minced ginger

3 medium garlic cloves, minced, or 1 tablespoon prepared minced garlic

1¼ cups vegetable broth

16 seedless white grapes, halved

1 pound (about 30) peeled, deveined medium shrimp,

DIRECTIONS

1. Mix the salt, dry mustard, coriander, cumin, ginger, turmeric, cayenne, cinnamon, and cloves in a small bowl. Stir in the vinegar to make a paste. Set aside.

2. Spray a large saucepan with nonstick cooking spray; set over medium heat for 1 minute. Add the onion; cook, stirring often, until softened, about 4 minutes.

3. Add the ginger and garlic; cook for 20 seconds. Add the spice paste; cook for 30 seconds, until aromatic. Stir in broth and

(*continued on next page*)

Shrimp Vindaloo (*cont.*)

grapes. Reduce the heat to medium-low and simmer, uncovered, for 10 minutes.

4. Add the shrimp, raise the heat to medium-high, and cook for 4 minutes, until the shrimp are pink and firm.

YIELD: 4 servings

TIPS: Vindaloo is usually served over rice because the starch cuts the heat. You can use brown rice here. However, it's just as good over a bed of cucumber noodles. Simply use a vegetable peeler to create long, thin noodles from peeled cucumbers, stopping when you get to the seedy core.

To save a little time, omit the first 9 ingredients; use 1 tablespoon Madras curry powder, or another hot curry powder, and mix the red-wine vinegar into it. (Vindaloo curry powder is very hard to find and often unbalanced in flavor.) You may need to add salt to taste at the end of the recipe if the curry powder you use doesn't include salt.

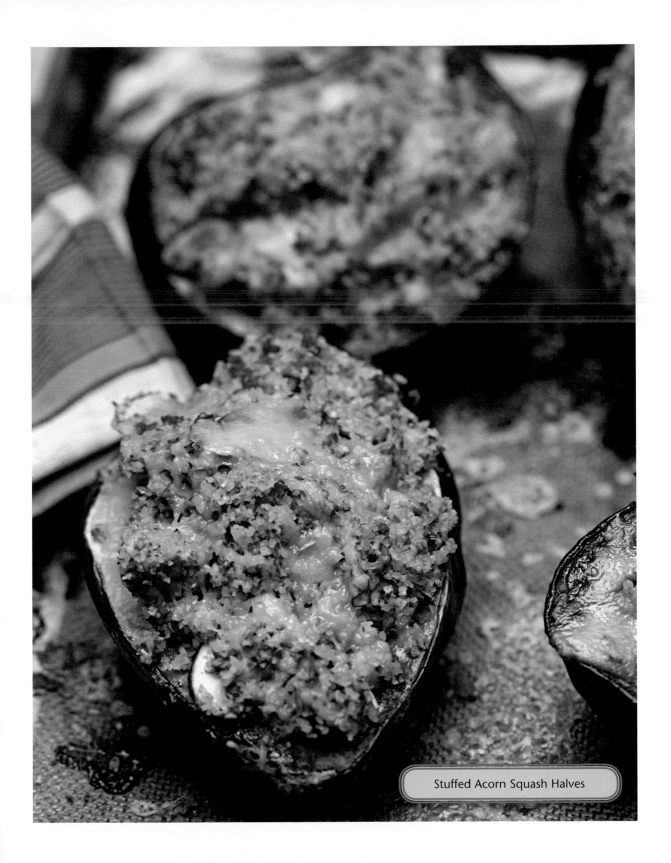

Stuffed Acorn Squash Halves

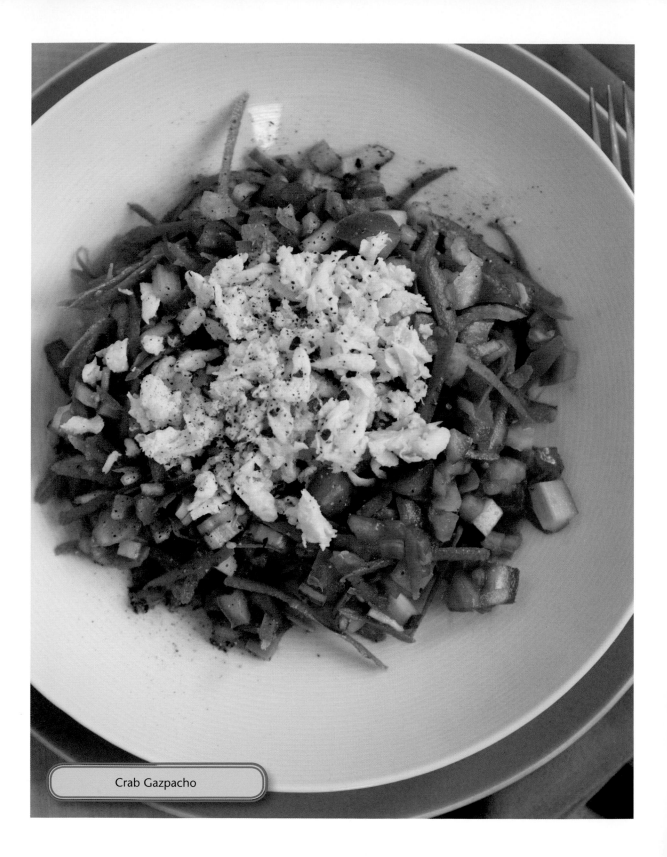

Crab Gazpacho

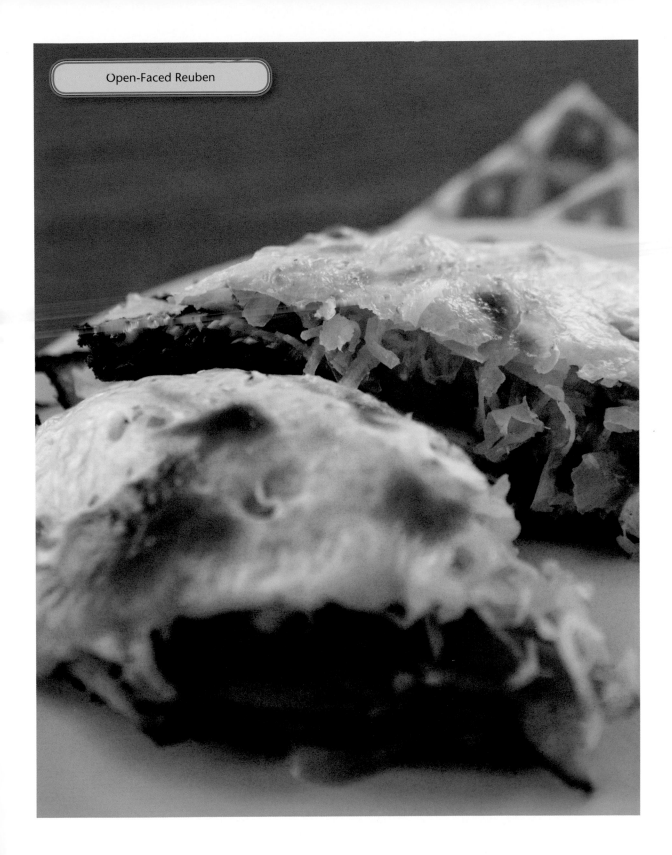

Open-Faced Reuben

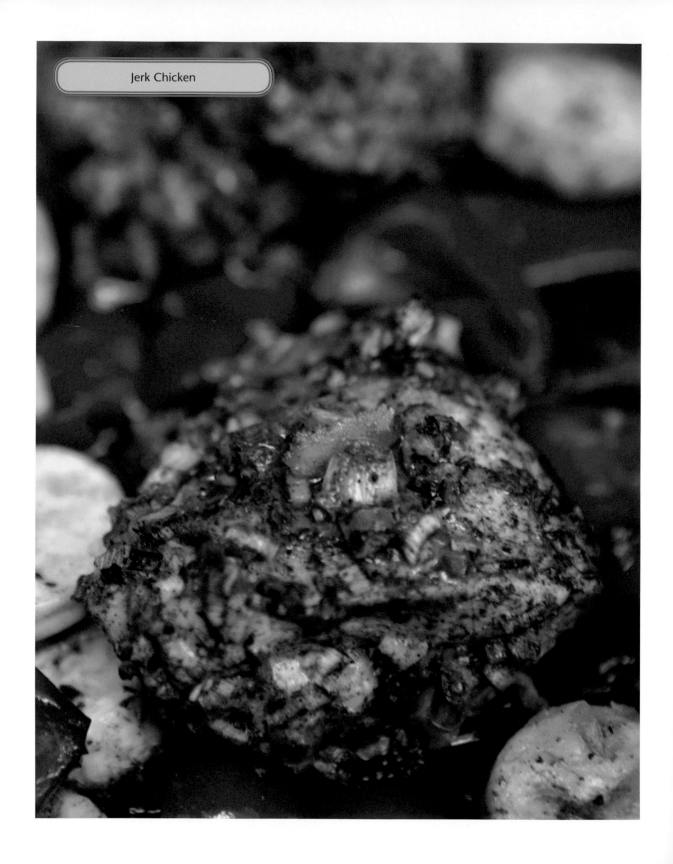

Jerk Chicken

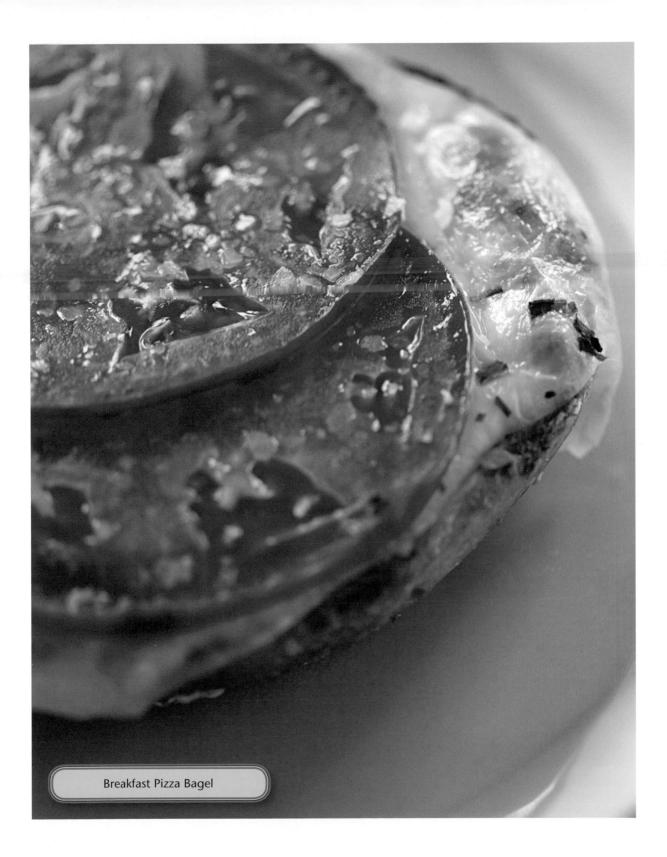

Breakfast Pizza Bagel

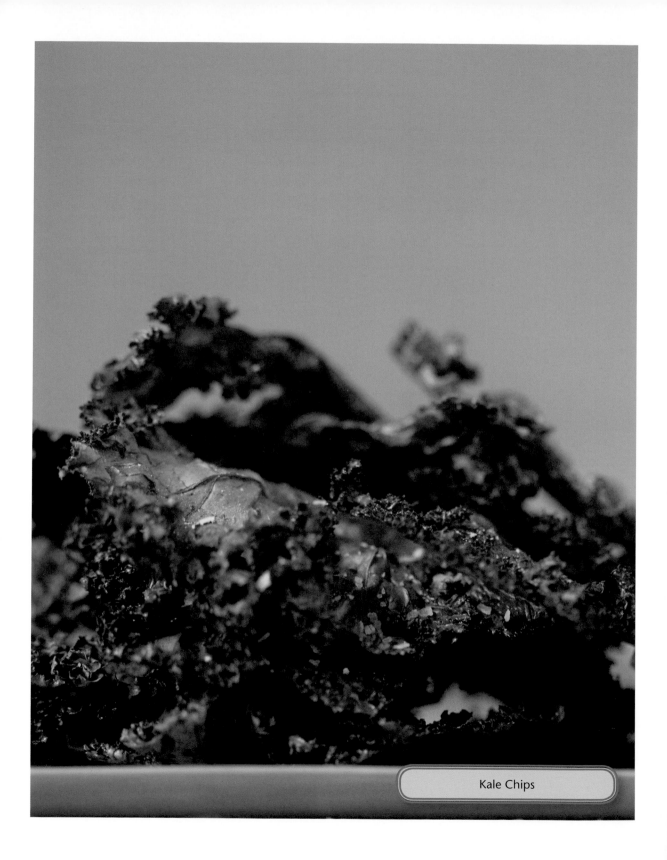

Kale Chips

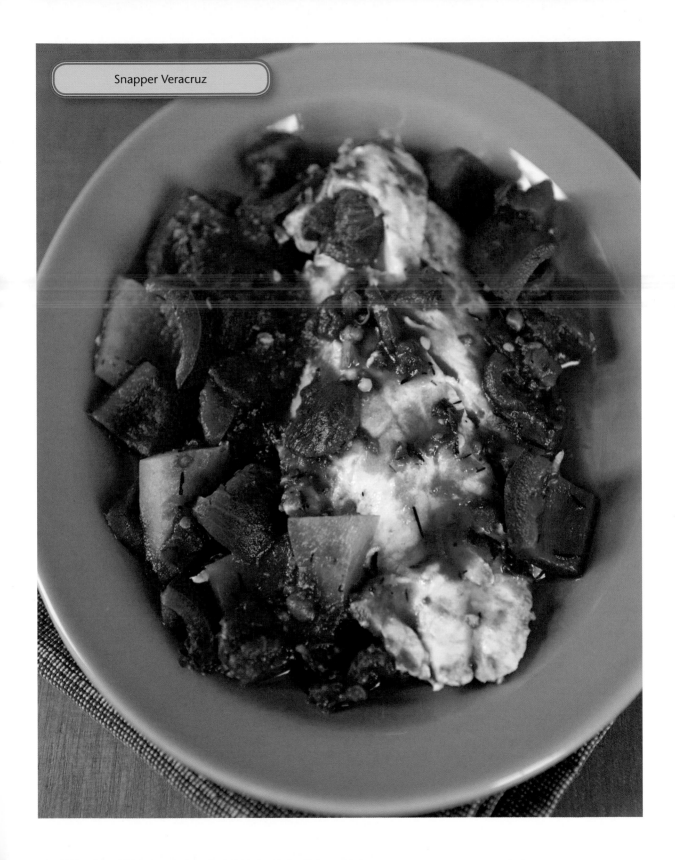

Snapper Veracruz

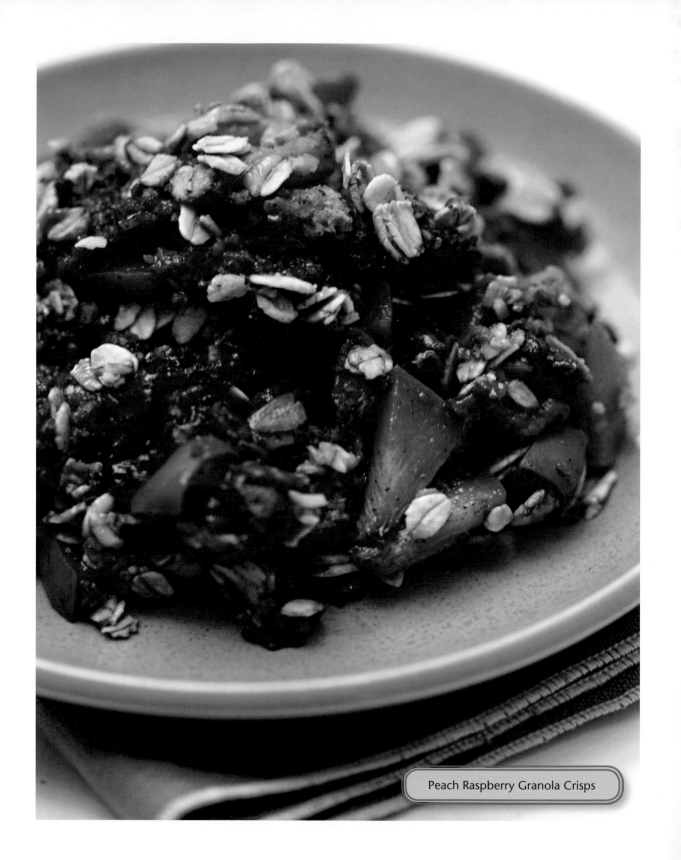

Peach Raspberry Granola Crisps

Arroz con Game Hens

Ask a Latin-American like me where to find a good arroz con pollo recipe and the answer is usually: "At my mom's." Arroz con pollo (rice with chicken) is a hearty, satisfying, inexpensive dish that's a meal in itself. It's usually made in one pan or a casserole on the stovetop, with chicken stock and spices added to the chicken's juices. Saffron turns the rice golden, and peas top the dish. It's easy and appealing, perfect for a healthy family dinner or for company. Here we make it with nutrient-packed brown rice and Cornish game hens, a flavorful, tender variation on a classic Latino dish.

INGREDIENTS

- 1 tablespoon olive oil
- Two 1-pound Cornish game hens, skinned and halved lengthwise
- 1 small yellow onion, chopped
- 1 medium green bell pepper, stemmed, seeded, and chopped
- 2 medium garlic cloves, minced, or 2 teaspoons prepared minced garlic
- 1 can (14 ounces) reduced sodium diced tomatoes, drained, juices reserved
- ¾ cup long-grain brown rice, such as brown basmati
- 2 teaspoons dried oregano
- ½ teaspoon ground allspice
- ½ teaspoon salt
- ½ teaspoon ground black pepper
- ¼ teaspoon saffron, optional
- 2 cups fat-free, low-sodium chicken broth
- 1 cup frozen green peas

DIRECTIONS

1. Heat the oil in a Dutch oven or a large pot. Put the game hens in the pot and brown on both sides, about 10 minutes, turning once. Transfer the game hens to a cutting board or a bowl.

(continued on next page)

Arroz con Game Hens (*cont.*)

2. Add the onion, bell pepper, and garlic to the pot; cook, stirring often, until softened, about 4 minutes. Pour in the diced tomatoes and all their juice; stir in the rice, oregano, allspice, salt, pepper, and saffron, if desired. Bring to a simmer, then stir over the heat until the tomatoes begin to break down, about 2 minutes.

3. Pour in the broth, nestle the game hens into the pot, and sprinkle the peas over the top. Cover, reduce the heat to low, and simmer until the rice is tender and the liquid is almost all absorbed, about 50 minutes. Set aside for 10 minutes to allow flavors to meld.

YIELD: 4 servings

TIPS: Ask a butcher at to skin and halve the game hens for you. Because of liquid content and cooking times, you can't use white rice with this dish. It has to be made with brown. You can use brown jasmine for a more aromatic dish. The secret to keeping the game hens from sticking is to let them, well, let them brown and keep going, undisturbed. They'll brown, caramelize, and then those natural sugars will release from the pot and you can pop the game hens off the bottom of the pot. Moving and nudging them starts the process all over with new sugars exposed, and more sticking.

Crab Cakes

It's not easy to downsize crab cakes into something you can enjoy while losing weight, but this recipe succeeds. With the addition of low-fat mayonnaise, they're moist and delicious with a perfect spicy tang. Using whole-wheat panko bread crumbs rather than cracker crumbs spikes up the nutrition.

INGREDIENTS

Nonstick cooking spray

½ small yellow onion, minced

1 celery stalk, minced

8 ounces pasteurized lump crabmeat

2 tablespoons low-fat mayonnaise

2 tablespoons whole-wheat panko bread crumbs

1 tablespoon Dijon mustard

1 teaspoon Cajun seasoning blend

¼ cup sugar-free cocktail sauce or calorie-free seafood sauce, such as Walden Farms

DIRECTIONS

1. Spray a large skillet, preferably nonstick, with nonstick cooking spray. Set over medium heat, then add the onion and celery. Cook, stirring often, until the onion softens, about 3 minutes. Transfer the vegetables to a large bowl; let cool for 5 minutes. Set skillet aside.

2. Add the crabmeat, mayonnaise, bread crumbs, mustard, and spice blend. Stir gently to create a uniform mixture. Divide into four even cakes, about ¾-inch thick, patting them between your palms to make sure they cohere.

3. Spray the skillet again with nonstick cooking spray; set over medium heat for 1 minute. Slip the crab cakes into the skillet and cook until brown and crunchy, about 8 minutes, turning once. Serve each cake with 1 tablespoon cocktail sauce.

YIELD: 4 servings

(continued on next page)

Crab Cakes (*cont.*)

TIPS: The trick here is to mince the celery as fine as possible so there are no chunks in the final cakes. Chopped celery from the refrigerator case in the produce section won't work unless you mince the bits more finely at home.

Also, don't use shelf-stable, canned crabmeat, found next to the canned tuna at the store. Search out the pasteurized containers at the fish counter of most supermarkets, usually in a refrigerator case. No need to buy jumbo lump or anything fancy like that since you're mixing it with other ingredients.

Oven-Fried Pork Chops

Few pork dishes are more delectable than pan-fried pork chops, but who needs all that fat? An alternative is oven-frying, in which you bread the chops with nutritious whole-wheat panko bread crumbs and use just a few sprays of nonstick cooking spray to impart a fried feel. Then bake and voilà *. . . I defy anyone to tell the difference.*

INGREDIENTS

Four 4-ounce center-cut boneless pork loin chops, about ½-inch thick

2 cups whole-wheat panko bread crumbs

1 tablespoon Italian seasoning blend

1½ cups low-fat buttermilk

Nonstick cooking spray

DIRECTIONS

1. Position a rack in the center of the oven; preheat to 400°F.

2. Trim any excess fat from the edges of the pork chops. Mix the bread crumbs and seasoning blend in a shallow bowl. Pour the buttermilk into a second shallow bowl

3. Spray a large baking pan with nonstick cooking spray. Dip one pork chop into the buttermilk, coating thoroughly on both sides. Hold the pork chop over the bowl for a moment to drain off any excess buttermilk. Set it in the bread crumbs; press these onto the chop on both sides. Transfer to the baking sheet. Repeat with the 3 remaining pork chops.

4. Spray the tops of the pork chops with nonstick cooking spray. Bake until browned and cooked through, about 15 minutes.

YIELD: 4 servings

Slow-Cooker Pulled Pork

Attention, barbecue lovers! That should be just about everyone. No longer is barbecue off limits while you're shedding pounds. Here's a recipe that has all the bold, meaty, tangy flavor you crave in a plate of great barbecued pork.

INGREDIENTS

1 large yellow onion, peeled and chopped

1 cup sugar-free, no-calorie barbecue sauce

1 tablespoon chili powder

One 2-pound boneless center-cut pork loin, trimmed of all surface fat

DIRECTIONS

1. Mix the onion, barbecue sauce, and chili powder in a 5- to 6-quart slow cooker. Nestle the pork loin in the sauce.

2. Cover and cook on low for 8 to 10 hours, until the pork is falling-apart tender. Shred the meat, using forks. Stir well to combine with the sauce.

YIELD: 8 servings

> **TIPS:** There are all sorts of sugar-free barbecue sauces from Walden Farms. The pulled pork freezes very well. Take the remaining servings and serve in individual containers so you can have a pulled pork lunch from the microwave anytime.

Lamb and Sweet Potato Stew

Preparing this tasty lamb stew is easy and not especially time consuming. Once it's on the table, you'll have a one-pot meal loaded with nutrition. Make sure you get your lamb well trimmed of all the white fat, because lamb can be on the fatty side.

INGREDIENTS

- 2 pounds lamb stew meat from the leg, cut into ½-inch pieces
- 2 pounds sweet potatoes, peeled and cut into thin spears
- 8 ounces thinly sliced white button mushrooms
- 4 large shallots, peeled and halved
- 8 whole garlic cloves, peeled
- 1 cup fat-free chicken broth
- 1 tablespoon sugar-free orange marmalade
- 2 teaspoons chopped fresh rosemary leaves or 1 teaspoon dried rosemary, crushed
- ½ teaspoon salt
- ½ teaspoon black pepper

DIRECTIONS

1. Place all the ingredients in a Dutch oven on the stovetop or in a 5- to 6-quart slow cooker; stir until well combined.

2. If using a Dutch oven, cover and bring to a simmer—then reduce the heat to low and cook until the meat and potatoes are tender, about 2½ hours. If using a slow cooker, cover and cook on low for 8 to 10 hours.

YIELD: 8 servings

> **TIP:** Have the butcher cube the meat from a boneless leg of lamb for you. This will makes life so much easier!

Polynesian London Broil

Ready for a big, beefy taste? Try this over-the-top recipe. London broil isn't tender like filet mignon. However, after a long bath in a pineapple, soy sauce, scallions, ginger, and garlic, even this rather tough slab of beef turns out a tender close second to a filet. Marinades like this one also add flavor to steak. Then get grilling! Can't you just hear the sizzle and smell that unmistakable grilled aroma?

INGREDIENTS

1 cup finely chopped fresh pineapple

½ cup light soy sauce

2 medium scallions, sliced thin

1 minced medium garlic clove or 1 teaspoon jarred minced garlic

1 tablespoon minced peeled fresh ginger or jarred minced ginger

1 teaspoon Truvia

Nonstick cooking spray

1½ pounds top round London broil

DIRECTIONS

1. Stir the pineapple, soy sauce, scallions, garlic, ginger, and Truvia in a medium bowl. Set the beef in a shallow baking dish and pour the pineapple mixture over the meat. Cover and refrigerate for at least 6 hours or overnight, turning occasionally.

2. Spray the grill rack or a grill pan with cooking spray. Prepare the grill for direct, high-heat cooking or heat the grill pan over medium-high heat. Place the London broil on the grill rack directly over the heat or in the grill pan. Cook, basting often with the remaining marinade and fruit in the baking dish, until desired degree of doneness, about 12 minutes for medium rare, about 14 minutes for medium. Transfer to a carving board and let stand for 5 minutes. Cut steak diagonally across grain into thin slices.

YIELD: 6 servings

TIP: To discover the grain of a steak for carving it properly, run your fingers across its surface. You'll see the grain open up, about like the grain of wood. For the most tender cuts, slice the steak diagonally across that grain.

Beef Barley Soup

I love this soup, especially on wintry nights. It's so easy to fix. All you have to do is toss the ingredients in a saucepan. The hard part is waiting two hours until it's ready! You'll be serving up a filling bowl of nutrition, too. Barley is one of the highest fiber grains you can eat, and fiber is a fat-burner.

INGREDIENTS

¾ pound beef sirloin, trimmed and cut into ½-inch pieces

6 cups fat-free beef broth

6 ounces white button mushrooms, sliced thin

1 medium yellow onion, chopped

1 large carrot, sliced thin

2 celery ribs, sliced thin

⅔ cup quick-cooking barley

1 tablespoon fresh thyme leaves or 1½ teaspoons dried thyme

½ teaspoon salt

½ teaspoon ground black pepper

1 bay leaf

Several dashes hot red-pepper sauce, optional

DIRECTIONS

1. Combine the beef, broth, mushrooms, onion, carrot, celery, barley, thyme, salt, pepper, and bay leaf in a large saucepan; bring to a full simmer over medium-high heat, stirring occasionally.

2. Cover, reduce the heat to low, and simmer slowly until beef is tender, about 2 hours, stirring once in a while. Discard the bay leaf and stir in hot red-pepper sauce, if desired, before serving.

YIELD: 4 servings

Jerk Chicken

A Jamaica-derived dish, true jerk chicken takes hours of slow cooking, but you can get a hint of the flavor, and a great meal, by rubbing the chicken with the spices listed here. Note that the recipe includes plantains, *which are close cousins to bananas, and a nutrition-packed alternative to rice and other starches. A cup of plantain supplies nearly half your daily vitamin C requirement, more than a third of the vitamin A, and provides three grams of fiber.*

INGREDIENTS

4 medium scallions, minced

1 small fresh jalapeño pepper, stemmed, seeded, and minced

1 tablespoon apple-cider vinegar

2 teaspoons minced peeled fresh ginger or jarred minced ginger

1 minced medium garlic clove or 1 teaspoon jarred minced garlic

1 teaspoon olive oil

1 teaspoon Truvia

½ teaspoon ground allspice

½ teaspoon ground coriander

½ teaspoon dried thyme

½ teaspoon ground cinnamon

½ teaspoon salt

½ teaspoon ground black pepper

Three ½-pound bone-in skinless chicken breasts, cut in half across

1 plantain, peeled and sliced

1 medium red bell pepper, stemmed, seeded, and coarsely chopped

DIRECTIONS

1. Mix the scallions, jalapeño, vinegar, ginger, garlic, oil, Truvia, allspice, coriander, thyme, cinnamon, salt, and pepper in a small bowl.

(continued on next page)

Jerk Chicken (*cont.*)

2. Place the chicken in a 9- x 13-inch baking dish; use a rubber spatula to spread the jerk marinade over the pieces. Sprinkle the plantain and bell pepper pieces around the baking dish. Cover with aluminum foil and refrigerate for at least 2 hours or up to 6 hours.

3. Position a rack in the center of the oven and preheat to 375°F.

4. Bake, covered, for 15 minutes. Uncover and continue baking until the chicken is cooked through and the plantains are tender, about 20 more minutes.

YIELD: 4 servings

> **TIPS:** To save time, use ⅓ cup wet jerk seasoning rub instead of making your own spice blend. Do not use a dry spice blend. You want the wet stuff.
>
> For way more heat and even a more authentic taste, substitute 1 stemmed, seeded, and minced habanero chili for the jalapeño chili.
>
> When working with hot chilies, wear rubber gloves to avoid burns. Failing that, rub your hands thoroughly with olive oil before you wash them to dissolve the chemical that causes the hot burn. Don't touch your eyes, ears, mouth, or any sensitive bits with unwashed hands.

Chicken and Apricot Sauté

If your attempts to eat lean and get lean have left you bored with skinless chicken breasts, the Chicken and Apricot Sauté below will be a tasty pleasant surprise, and it is so quick to fix. The breasts are sautéed, then doused with a warm apricot sauce that introduces a new dimension to the dish. Among fruits, apricots are among the highest in health-boosting antioxidants.

INGREDIENTS

Four 4-ounce boneless skinless chicken breasts

½ teaspoon salt

½ teaspoon ground black pepper

1 tablespoon olive oil

½ small red onion, chopped

4 medium apricots, pitted and sliced thin

½ cup fat-free chicken broth

2 teaspoons fresh thyme leaves or 1 teaspoon dried thyme

2 teaspoons apple-cider vinegar

DIRECTIONS

1. Season the chicken breasts with salt and pepper.

2. Heat ½ tablespoon olive oil in a large skillet, preferably nonstick. Add the chicken; cook until brown and cooked through, about 8 minutes, turning once. Transfer the chicken breasts to four serving plates or a serving platter.

3. Add the remaining ½ tablespoon oil to the skillet. Add the onion and apricot slices; cook, stirring almost constantly, for 2 minutes. Stir in the broth and thyme; bring to a full boil. Boil for 1 minute. Stir in the vinegar, boil for 30 seconds, and spoon the sauce over the chicken breasts.

YIELD: 4 servings

TIP: Substitute walnut oil or almond oil for the olive oil, for a subtle change in flavor.

Turkey and Mushroom Sloppy Joes

How's this for luscious and low-fat? Ounce for ounce, turkey breast yields less dietary fat than chicken breast or any cut of the leanest beef. Four ounces weighs in with a single gram of fat and a whopping 26 grams of protein. In these oh-so-delicious Sloppy Joes, we've taken the fat and calories down a few more notches by replacing some of the meatiness with meaty-tasting mushrooms.

INGREDIENTS

1¼ pounds white button or cremini mushrooms, sliced thin

1 tablespoon olive oil

12 ounces lean ground turkey

1 medium yellow onion, chopped

3 medium garlic cloves, minced, or 1 tablespoon prepared minced garlic

2 tablespoons balsamic vinegar

2 tablespoons Worcestershire sauce

1 tablespoon minced fresh oregano or 1½ teaspoons dried oregano

½ cup tomato paste

2 tablespoons calorie-free barbecue sauce, such as Waldens

½ teaspoon salt

½ teaspoon ground black pepper

4 slices whole-grain toast

DIRECTIONS

1. Place the mushrooms in a food processor fitted with the chopping blade. Process until ground to the consistency of ground beef.

2. Heat the oil in a large saucepan over medium heat. Add ground turkey; cook, stirring often, until it loses its raw, pink color, about 4 minutes.

3. Add mushrooms, onion, and garlic. Continue cooking, stirring often, until onions soften and mushrooms give off most of their liquid, about 3 minutes. Stir in the vinegar, Worcestershire, and oregano; simmer for 1 minute.

4. Stir in the tomato paste, barbecue sauce, salt, and pepper. Cook, stirring constantly to prevent scorching, until thick, to the point at which the mixture will hold its shape on a spoon, about 8 minutes. Serve open-faced on toast.

YIELD: 4 servings

> **TIP:** It's important to have those mushrooms really finely minced. If you don't own a food processor, you can put the mushrooms on a cutting board and rock a large knife through them repeatedly, slowly grinding/mincing them to the desired consistency. You really have to go at it. Even when you think it's finely minced, do some more work with the knife, just to be sure.

Stuffed Acorn Squash Halves

Here's a novel, scrumptious way to prepare acorn squash, a treat that earns its keep as a nutrient-rich veggie. A typical serving of acorn squash provides about 40 percent of the adult daily requirement for vitamin A, as well as contributing B vitamins, and some iron and other minerals. It is also a fairly rich source of potassium. This dish makes a tasty complement to just about any meat entrée.

INGREDIENTS

Nonstick cooking spray

2 medium acorn squash, halved and seeds and membranes removed

1 cup quick-cooking bulgur

4 ounces reduced-fat turkey sausage meat, crumbled

8 ounces white button or cremini mushrooms, sliced thin

1 tablespoon Italian seasoning blend

2 tablespoons sweet chili sauce

¼ cup grated low-fat cheddar cheese

DIRECTIONS

1. Position a rack in the center of the oven and preheat to 350°F.

2. Spray a 9- x 13-inch baking dish with cooking spray. Set the squash halves, cut side down, in the dish. Bake until tender when pierced through the skin with a knife, about 45 minutes.

3. Meanwhile, bring 1½ cups water to a boil in a small saucepan over high heat. Stir in the bulgur; cover and set aside off the heat for 30 minutes or until all the water has been absorbed.

4. Spray a large skillet with cooking spray and set over medium heat. Add the sausage; cook, stirring often, until browned, about 5 minutes.

5. Add the mushrooms; cook, stirring occasionally, until they give off their liquid, about 5 more minutes. Stir in the bulgur, seasoning blend, and chili sauce. Stir until uniform.

6. Once the squash halves are tender, use heat-safe oven mitts or two spatulas or tongs to turn them over without piercing them. Divide the turkey mixture between the halves, filling the cavities. Top each with 1 tablespoon cheese. Bake until the cheese has melted and browned a bit, about 10 minutes. Cool for 5 minutes before serving.

YIELD: 4 servings

TIPS: Substitute crumbled soy sausage, if you'd like. Scrub the squash really well. When tender, the skin is edible.

Amaranth Polenta

Polenta is usually made with cornmeal, but you can make it with amaranth, too. On its way to being a household word, amaranth is a whole grain that offers something processed grains don't: lots of high-quality protein. It's also a natural source of fiber, iron, calcium, and phosphorous.

INGREDIENTS

2 teaspoons olive oil

2 medium shallots, peeled, halved, and sliced thin

6 ounces white button or cremini mushrooms, sliced thin

1½ cups vegetable broth

1 cup whole-grain amaranth

1 teaspoon dried thyme

½ teaspoon salt

½ teaspoon black pepper

2 tablespoons finely grated Parmigiano-Reggiano

DIRECTIONS

1. Heat the oil in a medium saucepan over medium heat. Add the shallots; cook, stirring often, until softened, about 2 minutes. Add the mushrooms; cooking, stirring occasionally, until they give off their liquid and it coats the pan, about 2 minutes.

2. Stir in the broth, amaranth, thyme, salt, and pepper. Raise the heat to medium-high and bring to a full boil. Cover, reduce the heat to low, and simmer until thick and polentalike, about 30 minutes, stirring several times. Stir in cheese.

YIELD: 4 servings

TIPS: Be sure to use whole-grain amaranth, such as Arrowhead Mills Organic Whole Grain Amaranth, not amaranth grits. You can find it at large supermarkets in the organic aisle or at health-food stores. It cooks into something sort of like polenta but stickier. And it will firm up if you don't eat it pretty quickly, say, within 10 minutes. So, you can't make it ahead and set it on the back of the stove. Still, it makes a great side dish!

Zucchini, Lemon, and Parmesan Sauté

In France and Great Britain, zucchini is referred to as courgettes, *which has more to do with its scientific name Curcurbita than its historical heritage. Italians brought this tasty veggie and its name, zucchino, with them to America in the early twentieth century. It's so versatile that you can eat it raw, add it to salads, steam it, boil it, bake it, stuff it, and more. Here we sauté it. When it comes to nutrition, zucchini is great. A cup of sliced zucchini is packed with vitamin C and supplies only 16 calories.*

INGREDIENTS

2 medium zucchini

Nonstick cooking spray

½ teaspoon salt

Finely grated zest from 1 medium lemon

¼ cup sliced almonds, toasted

3 tablespoons finely grated Parmigiano-Reggiano

½ teaspoon ground black pepper

DIRECTIONS

1. Shred the zucchini through the large holes of a box grater and into a large bowl. Squeeze handfuls of the zucchini shreds over the sink to remove excess moisture.

2. Spray a large skillet with cooking spray and set over medium heat for 1 minute. Add the zucchini; cook, stirring often, until wilted, about 2 minutes. Stir in the salt and lemon zest; continue to stir over the heat for 1 minute.

3. Remove the skillet from the heat. Stir in the almonds and cheese. Top with pepper and serve.

YIELD: 4 servings

TIP: To toast sliced almonds, put them in a dry skillet over low heat and cook about 3 minutes, stirring occasionally. You can sometimes find toasted almonds on the salad bar at the supermarket.

Kale Chips

All hail, kale chips! You'll no longer need to worry about satisfying cravings for fattening potato chips once you've tried these. Crunch a few and you'll never have your hand in a bag of chips again, or at least I hope not!

INGREDIENTS

1 pound kale leaves, washed and dried
Nonstick cooking spray
½ teaspoon salt

DIRECTIONS

1. Position the racks in the top and bottom thirds of the oven; pre-heat to 375°F.

2. Cut out the thick, center stems from the kale leaves; tear the leaves themselves into ragged 3-inch pieces.

3. Spray two large baking sheets with nonstick cooking spray. Lay the leaf pieces on them in a single layer. Spray the leaves lightly with nonstick cooking spray.

4. Set the trays on the two racks. Bake for 15 minutes. Use tongs to turn the leaves over; reverse the trays top to bottom. Continue baking until crisp, about 15 more minutes. Sprinkle with salt while hot.

YIELD: 4 servings

TIP: Make sure the kale leaves are completely dry before you start this recipe.

Three Popcorn Spice Mixes

Popcorn is one of the healthiest snacks around. It's low in calories (about 23 calories per cup) and high in fiber. Only when soaked in butter and showered in salt does it become fattening. Because of this, most of us try to eat popcorn plain. However, there are other ways to enjoy it; here's how to spice up your popcorn experience.

INGREDIENTS

Parmesan and Herb

⅓ cup finely grated Parmigiano-Reggiano
½ teaspoon dried thyme
½ teaspoon dried oregano
½ teaspoon dried basil
½ teaspoon salt
½ teaspoon ground black pepper

Curried Cheddar

⅓ cup finely grated low-fat Cheddar
½ teaspoon curry powder
½ teaspoon onion powder
½ teaspoon salt
¼ teaspoon garlic powder

Cajun Spice

2 teaspoons mild paprika
½ teaspoon dried thyme
½ teaspoon onion powder
½ teaspoon celery seeds
½ teaspoon salt
¼ teaspoon garlic powder
¼ teaspoon cayenne

(continued on next page)

Three Popcorn Spice Mixes (*cont.*)

DIRECTIONS

To make spiced popcorn, put 4 cups popped popcorn in a large bowl; spray lightly with vegetable cooking spray. Mix one of the spice blends in a small bowl and sprinkle over the popcorn. Toss well.

YIELD: 4 servings

> **TIP:** Use real Parmigiano-Reggiano for recipes and shred it yourself with the small holes of a box grater or a microplane. The grated Parmesan in cans is often made with lots of oils and chemical fillers. Better to buy a chunk of this cheese and keep it tightly wrapped in the fridge until you need it.

Stuffed Figs

Here's a fig deal for you: scrumptiously stuffed figs that taste every bit as yummy as pieces of chocolate candy. Figs are loaded with magnesium, calcium, potassium, even a little protein and zinc. The biggest nutrition bonanza in this fruit is its fiber. So many people take laxatives, but if they had more figs in their diet, they wouldn't need them.

INGREDIENTS

4 large figs

2 ounces soft, fresh goat cheese (chèvre)

¼ teaspoon ground black pepper

4 walnut halves

¼ cup sugar free chocolate sauce

DIRECTIONS

Split each fig from the stem down without cutting all the way through to the bottom. Open the slit a bit and spread ½ ounce goat cheese inside the fig. Sprinkle the cheese with black pepper; place a walnut half in each fig. Set the figs on serving plates and drizzle each with 1 tablespoon chocolate sauce.

YIELD: 4 servings

TIP: For more flavor, toast the walnut halves in a dry skillet for a couple of minutes and cool completely before using. Sugar-free chocolate sauces vary in flavor and goodness; one of the most delicious sugar-free chocolate sauces is made by Smucker's.

Peach Raspberry Granola Crisps

This recipe is a take on traditional fruit cobbler, only healthier and virtually fat free. It's even okay to serve it for breakfast.

INGREDIENTS

Nonstick cooking spray

1 large peach, pitted and chopped

1½ cups raspberries

2 tablespoons whole-wheat panko bread crumbs

2 teaspoons Truvia

½ teaspoon ground cinnamon

1 cup low-fat granola

DIRECTIONS

1. Position a rack in the center of the oven and preheat to 350°F.

2. Spray 4 cups in a muffin tin with cooking spray. Mix the peaches, raspberries, bread crumbs, Truvia, and cinnamon in a bowl; divide among the cups in the tin. Top each with ¼ cup granola.

3. Bake until bubbling and hot, about 30 minutes. Cool for 5 minutes in the tin before scooping into bowls.

YIELD: 4 servings

TIPS: To save time, use 1 cup of chopped, thawed, frozen sliced peaches. The granola should be fairly plain, without dried fruit, for example. You don't want any complicated flavors to compete with the peaches and raspberries.

Baked Bananas

Bananas alone make a great dessert, but wait until you liven them up like this! Yummy and full of nutrition, they're a great way to get your fat-burning probiotics in.

INGREDIENTS

Nonstick cooking spray

4 large bananas, peeled

¼ cup no-sugar-added apricot preserves or all-fruit spread

1 teaspoon vanilla extract

¼ teaspoon ground cinnamon

½ cup sugar-free, low-fat, vanilla yogurt or Greek yogurt

DIRECTIONS

1. Position a rack in the center of the oven and preheat to 400°F.

2. Lightly spray the inside of a small baking pan with nonstick cooking spray. Set the bananas in the pan. Spread the preserves over the bananas; sprinkle with the vanilla and cinnamon. Cover the baking dish with foil; bake for 20 minutes. Scoop the bananas and sauce onto plates; top each serving with 2 tablespoons yogurt.

YIELD: 4 servings

> **TIPS:** Make that the foil is sealed tightly. You can also use peach all-fruit spread, if desired, or even a sugar-free fig spread.

Grilled Pineapple with
Vanilla Ricotta and Pistachios

Think of this dessert as a pineapple sundae, because that's what it tastes like. I don't want to spoil that image for you, but the doctor in me does have to add something about how healthy this recipe is: full of protein, calcium, fiber, and natural enzymes.

INGREDIENTS

Nonstick cooking spray

1 large pineapple, peeled, cored, and chopped into 1-inch-thick spears

2 cups low-fat ricotta

2 teaspoons Truvia

2 teaspoons vanilla extract

½ cup shelled, chopped pistachios

DIRECTIONS

1. Spray a grill rack or a grill pan with nonstick cooking spray. Prepare the grill for direct, high-heat cooking; or heat the grill pan over medium-high heat until smoking.

2. Set the pineapple spears on the grill grate directly over the heat or in the grill pan. Grill until marked and hot, about 4 minutes, turning once. Divide the spears among four plates.

3. Mix the ricotta, Truvia, and vanilla in a small bowl. Dollop ½ cup on top of the grilled pineapple on each plate. Sprinkle with chopped pistachios.

YIELD: 4 servings

> **TIP:** You can often find a whole peeled, cored pineapple in the refrigerator case of the produce section, often sealed in a plastic container. You simply cut the pineapple into spears.

17 Sample Cycle 3 Menus

Here are examples of how to build menus using the preceding recipes while on the Achieve Cycle. You can follow these menus exactly or create your own.

Day 1

Breakfast

☐ 1 serving *Better Migas*

☐ ½ grapefruit, or other fresh fruit

☐ 1 cup green tea

Lunch

☐ 1 serving *Spinach Mushroom Salad with Warm Bacon Dressing*

☐ 1 serving fresh fruit

☐ 1 cup green tea

Dinner

☐ 1 serving *Slow-Cooker Pulled Pork*

☐ 1–2 cups tossed mixed salad with 2 tablespoons fat-free dressing

☐ 1 cup green tea

Snacks

☐ 1 probiotic, dairy, or dairy substitute serving

☐ 1 frozen fruit bar

Day 2

Breakfast

☐ 1 cup high-fiber cereal, such as Bran Buds or Fiber One

☐ 1 cup skim, 1%, or soy milk or other dairy substitute

☐ 1 cup fresh berries

☐ 1 cup green tea

Lunch

☐ 1 serving *White Bean and Oat Burgers*

☐ 10 baby carrots

☐ 1 cup green tea

Dinner

☐ 1 serving *Jerk Chicken*

☐ Steamed vegetables such as asparagus, wax beans, broccoli, or cauliflower

☐ 1 cup green tea

Snacks

☐ 1 serving *Stuffed Figs*

☐ 1 Skinny Cow ice-cream sandwich

Day 3

Breakfast

☐ 1 serving *Banana Chocolate Smoothie*

☐ 1 slice cracked-wheat toast

☐ 1 cup green tea

Lunch

☐ 1 serving *Crab Gazpacho*

☐ 1 cup green tea

Dinner

☐ 1 serving *Lamb and Sweet Potato Stew*

☐ 1 cup green tea

Snacks

☐ 1 serving *Baked Bananas*

☐ 2nd probiotic, dairy, or dairy substitute serving

Day 4

Breakfast

- ☐ 1 *Dr. Mike's Power Cookie*
- ☐ 1 cup skim, 1%, or soy milk or other dairy substitute
- ☐ 1 cup fresh berries
- ☐ 1 cup green tea

Lunch

- ☐ 1 serving *Shrimp Soba Noodle Salad*
- ☐ 1 medium apple or pear
- ☐ 1 cup green tea

Dinner

- ☐ 1 bowl *Beef Barley Soup*
- ☐ 1 cup green tea

Snacks

- ☐ 2nd probiotic, dairy, or dairy substitute serving
- ☐ *Kale Chips*

Day 5

Breakfast

- ☐ 2 scrambled eggs
- ☐ 1 serving *Slow-Cooker Brown Rice Congee*
- ☐ 1 cup fresh berries
- ☐ 1 cup green tea

Lunch

- ☐ 1 serving *Easy Cioppino*
- ☐ 1 fresh pear
- ☐ 1 cup green tea

Dinner

- ☐ 1 serving *Oven-Fried Pork Chops*
- ☐ Steamed broccoli
- ☐ 1–2 cups tossed mixed salad with 2 tablespoons fat-free dressing
- ☐ 1 cup green tea

Snacks

- ☐ Probiotic, dairy, or dairy substitute serving
- ☐ 1 100-calorie Fudgsicle

Day 6

Breakfast

☐ 1 cup sugar-free fruit-flavored yogurt

☐ ½ cup low-fat granola

☐ 1 piece fresh fruit (i.e., 1 peach, ¼ cantaloupe, ½ grapefruit, or 1 orange)

☐ 1 cup green tea

Lunch

☐ 1 serving *Crab Cakes*

☐ Medium baked potato with 1 tablespoon fat-free sour cream; or ½ cup brown or basmati rice

☐ 1 medium apple

☐ 1 cup green tea

Dinner

☐ 1 serving *Polynesian London Broil*

☐ Yellow squash, steamed

☐ 1 cup green tea

Snack

☐ 2nd probiotic, dairy, or dairy substitute serving

☐ 1 frozen fruit bar

Day 7

Breakfast

☐ 1 serving *Grilled Pineapple with Vanilla Ricotta and Pistachios*

☐ 1 cup green tea

Lunch

☐ 1 serving *Tex-Mex Millet Salad*

☐ 1 cup green tea

Dinner

☐ 1 serving *Roasted Trout Almandine*

☐ Steamed vegetables

☐ 1–2 cups tossed mixed salad with 2 tablespoons reduced-fat dressing

☐ 1 cup green tea

Snacks

☐ 6-ounces plain or sugar-free fruit-flavored yogurt

☐ 1 serving fresh fruit, in season

Day 8

Breakfast

☐ 1 *Dr. Mike's Power Cookie*

☐ 1 banana, sliced

☐ 1 cup nonfat or acidophilus milk

☐ 1 cup green tea

Lunch

☐ 1 serving *Brie and Mango Quesadilla*

☐ Spinach, steamed

☐ 1 cup green tea

Dinner

☐ 1 serving *Broiled Miso-Glazed Salmon*

☐ 1 serving *Stuffed Acorn Squash Halves*

☐ 1 cup green tea

Snacks

☐ 1 probiotic, dairy, or dairy substitute serving

☐ 1 frozen fruit bar

Day 9

Breakfast

- ☐ 1 serving *Breakfast Pizza Bagels*
- ☐ 1 cup fresh berries
- ☐ 1 cup green tea

Lunch

- ☐ 1 serving *Open-Faced Reuben*
- ☐ 1 cup green tea

Dinner

- ☐ 1 serving *Chicken and Apricot Sauté*
- ☐ Steamed vegetables such as asparagus, wax beans, broccoli, or cauliflower
- ☐ 1 cup green tea

Snacks

- ☐ *Kale Chips*
- ☐ 1 Skinny Cow ice-cream sandwich

Day 10

Breakfast

- ☐ ½ cup cooked oatmeal
- ☐ ½ grapefruit
- ☐ 1 cup green tea

Lunch

- ☐ 1 serving *Crab Gazpacho*
- ☐ 1 cup green tea

Dinner

- ☐ 1 serving *Turkey and Mushroom Sloppy Joes*
- ☐ 1–2 cups tossed mixed salad with 2 tablespoons reduced-fat dressing
- ☐ 1 cup green tea

Snacks

- ☐ 2nd fruit serving
- ☐ 2nd probiotic, dairy, or dairy substitute serving

Day 11

Breakfast

- ☐ 1 serving *Better Migas*
- ☐ 1 medium apple or pear
- ☐ 1 cup green tea

Lunch

- ☐ 1 serving *Crab Cakes*
- ☐ 1–2 cups tossed mixed salad with 2 tablespoons reduced-fat dressing
- ☐ 1 cup green tea

Dinner

- ☐ 1 serving *Snapper Veracruz*
- ☐ 1 serving *Peach Raspberry Granola Crisps*
- ☐ 1 cup green tea

Snacks

- ☐ 1 serving *Popcorn Spice Mix*
- ☐ 2nd probiotic, dairy, or dairy substitute serving

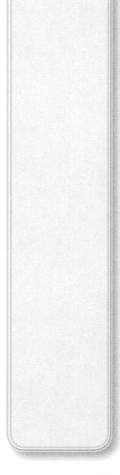

NOTES

Day 12

Breakfast

- ☐ 4 scrambled egg whites
- ☐ 1 slice Canadian bacon
- ☐ 1 cup melon balls
- ☐ 1 cup green tea

Lunch

- ☐ 1 serving *White Bean and Oat Burger*
- ☐ 1 fresh pear, or other fruit in season
- ☐ 1 cup green tea

Dinner

- ☐ 1 serving *Arroz con Game Hens*
- ☐ 1 cup green tea

Snacks

- ☐ Probiotic, dairy, or dairy-substitute serving
- ☐ 1 100-calorie Fudgsicle

Day 13

Breakfast

- ☐ 6 ounces sugar-free fruit-flavored yogurt
- ☐ 1 piece fresh fruit (i.e, 1 peach, ¼ cantaloupe, ½ grapefruit, or 1 orange)
- ☐ 1 cup green tea

Lunch

- ☐ 1 serving *Open-Faced Reuben*
- ☐ 1 medium apple
- ☐ 1 cup green tea

Dinner

- ☐ 4 to 6 ounces baked chicken breast
- ☐ 1 serving *Zucchini, Lemon, and Parmesan Sauté*
- ☐ 1 cup green tea

Snack

- ☐ 2nd probiotic, dairy, or dairy substitute serving
- ☐ 1 serving *Stuffed Figs*

Day 14

Breakfast

- ☐ 2 scrambled eggs
- ☐ 1 serving *Slow-Cooker Brown Rice Congee*
- ☐ 1 cup pineapple chunks, fresh or canned in their own juice
- ☐ 1 cup green tea

Lunch

- ☐ 1 serving *Brie and Mango Quesadilla*
- ☐ 1–2 cups tossed mixed salad with 2 tablespoons reduced-fat dressing
- ☐ 1 cup green tea

Dinner

- ☐ 1 serving *Slow-Cooker Pulled Pork*
- ☐ 1 cup of cole slaw tossed with low-fat cole-slaw dressing
- ☐ 1 cup green tea

Snack

- ☐ 2nd probiotic, dairy, or dairy substitute serving
- ☐ 1 medium orange

Day 15

Breakfast

- ☐ 1 serving *Banana Chocolate Smoothie*
- ☐ 1 cup green tea

Lunch

- ☐ 1 serving *Tex-Mex Millet Salad*
- ☐ 1 cup fresh berries
- ☐ 1 cup green tea

Dinner

- ☐ 1 serving *Shrimp Vindaloo*
- ☐ 1–2 cups tossed mixed salad with 2 tablespoons reduced-fat dressing
- ☐ 1 cup green tea

Snacks

- ☐ 1 probiotic, dairy, or dairy substitute serving
- ☐ 1 frozen fruit bar

NOTES

Day 16

Breakfast

- ☐ 1 cup high-fiber cereal, such as Bran Buds or Fiber One
- ☐ 1 cup skim, acidophilus, 1%, or soy milk or other dairy substitute
- ☐ 1 banana, sliced
- ☐ 1 cup green tea

Lunch

- ☐ 1 serving *Spinach Mushroom Salad with Warm Bacon Dressing*
- ☐ 1 cup green tea

Dinner

- ☐ 1 serving *Jerk Chicken*
- ☐ Steamed vegetables such as asparagus, wax beans, broccoli, or cauliflower
- ☐ 1 cup green tea

Snacks

- ☐ 2nd fruit serving
- ☐ 1 Skinny Cow ice-cream sandwich

Day 17

Breakfast

- ☐ 6 ounces nonfat Greek yogurt mixed with 1 tablespoon sugar-free jam
- ☐ 1 cup fresh berries
- ☐ 1 cup green tea

Lunch

- ☐ 1 serving *Crab Gazpacho*
- ☐ 1 cup green tea

Dinner

- ☐ 1 serving *Polynesian London Broil*
- ☐ 1 medium baked potato with 1 tablespoon reduced-fat sour cream or Greek yogurt
- ☐ 1–2 cups tossed mixed salad with 1 tablespoon oil mixed with 2 tablespoons vinegar
- ☐ 1 cup green tea

Snacks

- ☐ 2nd fruit serving
- ☐ 1 fat-free pudding cup

About Cycle 4: Arrive

After you have reached your goal weight by using Cycles 1 through 3 as directed, you graduate to Cycle 4: Arrive. This is the maintenance cycle of the 17 Day Diet. You fought the battle of the bulge and won. This is a huge, important accomplishment, something many people fail to do. Now, the important thing is that you stay at this weight.

Here's how you do that.

Enjoy yourself on the weekend. Yes, you can splurge on the weekends, if you'd like. Let's face it: Weekends have never been good for diets. You get a promotion on Friday, so you eat. Or you snuggle up to watch a movie on Friday or Saturday, and you eat. Or you go out to a party, and you eat. The problem is, from 6:00 P.M. on Friday until bedtime on Sunday, your life changes. Your schedule is looser, allowing for more snacking. Then there are the social commitments. Dinners out, birthday shindigs, Sunday brunch—they can do you in. It seems like you need thick layers of duct tape on your mouth to prevent pig-outs.

Taking weekends off allows you to splurge a bit, making it easier to get back on track on Monday. Most people can be pretty good Monday through Thursday, choosing meals carefully, getting in some exercise, and seeing decent results on the scale. The Arrive Cycle capitalizes on these normal rhythms of life and builds a *livable* maintenance plan around them.

Besides rapid weight loss, this is the feature of the 17 Day Diet everyone loves. Of course, come Monday morning, you simply minimize any overindulgent damage by getting back on one of the cycles.

Use your favorite cycle, and all your favorite recipes from this cookbook, during the week. On weekdays, stay strict and use your favorite cycle to control your weight. I'm giving you the best diet present you can have. You still eat a calorie-controlled diet during the week, then, on weekends, have what you'd like. You take off plenty of pounds, and you keep the weight off because you never get bored using my weekend principle.

The Arrive Cycle is metabolically strategic, too. You can control your weight efficiently because you're shocking your metabolism back into action. Why? Because you're following 5 days of controlled eating, followed by 2 days of increased calories. By adding calories to your meals with hamburgers, bread, ice cream, wine, cheesecake, you name it, you're speeding up your metabolism. Then, when your metabolism is roaring like a furnace, you get back to your diet on Monday, burning calories faster than ever. Basically, the Arrive Cycle keeps your metabolism guessing, so it never has a chance to go into hibernation. Since your metabolism is now well trained due to better eating habits and digestive health, a few cheat treats on the weekend will not have an adverse affect.

The Arrive Cycle is not a free-for-all, though. You're allowed some of your favorite foods in moderation. For example, Friday night: A restaurant meal with a cocktail or two at your favorite restaurant; Saturday: a slice or two of pizza for lunch or dinner, plus one dessert; Sunday: a breakfast of pancakes with maple syrup.

A good rule of thumb to follow while stabilizing your weight is to enjoy no more than one to three favorite meals each weekend. I call this *strategic cheating*. It works wonders for keeping weight off, and you'll love the freedom.

As a parting shot, let me say that millions of people have lost weight rapidly and safely on the 17 Day Diet. Now with *The 17 Day Diet Workbook* and *The 17 Day Cookbook*, you have more tools than ever to stick with this remarkably effective program.

What matters to me now is that you use the cookbook to help you arrive at your goal sooner than later. Try as many recipes as you can, pick your favorites, enjoy, and start loving your new, trimmer, shapelier physique.

Cheers . . . see you at your goal!

INDEX